Epidemiology for Field Veterinarians: An Introduction

Epidemiology for Field Veterinarians: An Introduction

Editor

Sharad Sawant

scitus
academics

Epidemiology for Field Veterinarians: An Introduction

Edited by **Sharad Sawant**

ISBN: 978-1-68117-059-6

Library of Congress Control Number: 2015935457

SCITUS Academics LLC,
www.scitusacademics.com
Box No. 4766, 616 Corporate Way,
Suite 2, Valley Cottage,
NY 10989

Printed in United States of America on Acid Free Paper ∞

Contents

Preface

Epizootiology, epizoology, or veterinary epidemiology is the study of disease patterns within animal populations. Veterinary epidemiology deals with the investigation of diseases, productivity and animal welfare in populations. It is used to describe the frequency of disease occurrence and how disease, productivity and welfare are affected by the interaction of different factors or determinants. Today, the veterinary profession is confronted with a different set of problems compared with the middle of last century. Now, veterinarians often have to deal with herds or regions remaining diseased after lengthy disease control campaigns. In addition, it is considered necessary to take into account the economic aspects of disease control through the use of benefit/cost analyses of disease control campaigns. Costly multi-factorial disease complexes such as mastitis or cattle lameness have become quite common. In addition, old, emerging or new diseases with complex aetiologies pose a difficult challenge for the profession. Veterinarians have to respond to the challenges posed by problems such as BSE, FMD and antimicrobial resistance. All these problems require identification, quantification and intensive examination of multiple, directly or indirectly causal, and often interacting, disease determinants. Veterinary epidemiology and evidence-based veterinary medicine provide overlapping sets of tools which can be used to approach these new challenges.

Editor

Chapter 1

The Material and Cultural Recovery of Camels and Camel Husbandry among Sahrawi Refugees of Western Sahara

Gabriele Volpato and Patricia Howard

Department of Social Sciences, Wageningen University, Hollandseweg 1, Wageningen 6706, KN, the Netherlands

ABSTRACT

For nearly 1,500 years, Sahrawi nomads of Western Sahara respected the camel; camels were essential to life in the desert environment, constituting both the main means of production and exchange and the keystone of Sahrawi cultural identity. The capacity to adapt to drought is crucial for the resilience of nomadic populations, which are particularly susceptible to its repeated occurrence. Knowledge of coping strategies is transmitted and embedded deeply within nomads' cultural institutions. In 1975, the Moroccan army occupied the Sahrawi's traditional nomadic territory, decimating camel herds and forcing most Sahrawi into refugee camps in Algeria where the Sahrawi became wholly dependent on foreign aid for their sustenance. However, with the signing of a ceasefire agreement in the early 1990s, the Sahrawi recovered part of their nomadic territory and the right to move within it, while at the same time, new flows of capital entered the camps. Refugees began to recover camel husbandry as a livelihood strategy and the camel re-emerged as a potent symbol as refugees and the Polisario Front (the Sahrawi's political representative) struggle to assert their new found national identity, regain access to all of their traditional territory and reaffirm their shared nomadic cultural heritage.

INTRODUCTION

For the past several decades, scholars and development organizations have increasingly focused on nomadic populations in part because, across the globe, their cultures and socio-ecological systems are threatened by the creation of political boundaries, forced sedentarization and resource depletion and in part because they have become aware of the complexity and efficacy of such systems in relation to resource management in harsh environmental conditions (Keenan[2003]; Gauthier-Pilters [1961]; Chatty [2005]). Research has also been conducted on the keystone role of the camel among these populations (Köhler-Rollefson [2003]), on their traditional ethnobiological and ethnoveterinary knowledge (Volpato et al. [2013a]; Mohamed and Hussein[1996]; Abbas et al. [2002]) and on the human-camel relations from an anthropological perspective (Catley [2006]).

Studies of herd loss and recovery among contemporary nomadic populations with drought and protracted conflict are central to pastoralist studies (Boneh [1984]; Khalif and Oba [2013]; Mezhoud and Oxby [2013]). Such studies are situated within an anthropological literature that understands sedentarization as a recurrent phenomenon within nomadic societies (Salzman[1980]; Adano and Witsenburg [2005]; Blench [2001]). The case of the Sahrawi can be contextualized precisely within this literature. Over the past 1,500 years, when their camel herds were largely depleted or severely weakened by drought or military assault, Sahrawi nomads could no longer appropriate desert resources and were forced to retreat to the periphery of their nomadic territories where they sought other means to survive outside of the desert, i.e. in oases, in coastal towns (where fishing was possible) or in agricultural settlements (Caro Baroja [1955]). Destitute nomads relocated to other areas either near wealthy camps or settlements (offering services to them, seeking assimilation and surviving on public slaughter and milk redistribution), or emigrating to the agricultural villages of the Oued Draa and Oued Nun or, less commonly, to the oases of central Mauritania. After herds were decimated by recurrent droughts, with the return of the rains, nomads began to repopulate the desert with their surviving herds or animals received in*mniha* (camel loans)[a]. Nomads who had lost all of their camels engaged in trade or other activities to acquire camels and initiate their real and metaphorical travel back towards the 'centre of the desert'.

Footnote

[a]Loans where those who borrow camels assume the costs of managing them and can use them for transport, milk production and wool.

In the 20th century, the strategies that the Sahrawi deploy to confront the Moroccan threat to their nomadic way of life and recover camels after dispossession while in exile in essence represent an extension or adaptation of their traditional mix of strategies for dealing with drought and military assault. In 1975, for the first time in their history, the Sahrawi were forced to confront an enemy with vastly superior military power and, in the process, lost all access to their traditional pastoral territories; most lost their mobility, herds and alternative means of livelihood. Most fled Morocco's military assaults, taking refuge in camps where they became utterly dependent upon foreign aid for the duration of the prolonged (16 years) guerrilla war that the Sahrawi waged against the Moroccan Army. The Sahrawi experienced greater social, cultural and political change living as refugees in a protracted situation. This time, the particular confluence of factors that permit refugees to proactively recover herds and reoccupy the desert, and the means by which they have adapted to these new conditions, signals profound changes in the economic, technical, social and cultural relations of camel husbandry in the Western Sahara and in the Sahrawi's social formation.

The study of pastoralists who have lost their herds and become refugees is directly relevant not only to the understanding of contemporary pastoralist societies that are confronted with herd loss and physical displacement, but as well to the study of refugees more generally and of their attempts to recover pre-conflict/pre-disaster livelihoods. Dispossessed pastoralists generally reconstitute herds only in the long term, which may be compared with the time required for refugees living in protracted situations to regain their subsistence strategies and cultural identity (Khalif and Oba [2013]; McCabe [1987]). In refugee camps, people's individual and collective agency - their capacity and actions to 'transcend the dictates of their immediate environment and... shape their life circumstances and the course of their lives' (Bandura [2006]. p. 165) - are severely constrained; they are deprived of access to most resources, confront limited opportunities (e.g. for mobility or education) and high levels of risk (e.g. looting, conflict, further displacement) (Jacobsen [2005]). When people become refugees, their traditional productive activities and the associated knowledge, cultural practices and artefacts may be lost forever. However, once in camps, as conditions permit, refugees struggle to reassert their agency, develop productive activities and revitalize the associated knowledge and practices. In the process, these are adapted to new environmental, social, cultural, political and economic contexts (Golooba-Mutebi and Tollman [2004]; Jacobsen [2002]; Horst [2006a]).

Because refugees lose everything with forced displacement into camps, recovery must occur from scratch. Studies about such autochthonous recovery processes (e.g. not purposively facilitated by aid agencies or governments) and of refugees' individual and collective agency can help to formulate policies that promote refugees' material and cultural well-being. The international community can support refugee's own efforts to regain access to the means of subsistence (e.g. livestock, land) by facilitating the economic means and necessary institutional conditions (e.g. mobility, security, legal entitlements) (Meyer [2006]). As the case study presented here shows, aid can be instrumental to the recovery process in that it represents a safety net for refugees who have no access to other resources, removes the burden of procuring basic provisions for survival while capitals are rebuilt and provides seed capital for refugees' own pursuits (Fiddian-Qasmiyeh [2011]; Lentz et al. [2005]). As Harvey and Lind ([2005], p. 26) argue for Turkana pastoralists of Kenya, 'Food aid can provide the incentive for pastoralists to hold onto animals, and thereby contribute to the livelihood recovery process after an emergency.'

As refugees' worldviews, beliefs, values, cognition (including knowledge) and social relations are strongly rooted in their pre-exile worlds, their recovery strategies are informed by pre-exile modes of subsistence, social relations, cultural values and adaptive strategies. Especially among former pastoral and nomadic refugees, and within the constraints presented by the structure of camps and access to pastoral territories, refugees' agency is directed towards the recovery of livestock husbandry, including a return, as far as possible, to nomadism or transhumance. At the same time, however, refugees become integrated within trans-regional and transnational processes through political struggles, foreign aid, emigration and informal and formal markets for wage labour and other commodities. Pastoralism and nomadism are also being transformed through economic globalization (Chatty [2005]; Bollig et al. [2013]; Gertel and Le Heron [2011]), and refugee herd recovery is thus accompanied by change in the material and cultural use and management of herds related to these larger transformation processes. The individual and collective struggles to recover pre-exile modes of subsistence and livestock husbandry are motivated not only by the desire to improve the material conditions of life and gain greater autonomy; pre-exile modes of subsistence have great continuing cultural significance that refugees and their political representatives may re-appropriate and adapt to promote and strengthen identity that underlie claims to national sovereignty and territory.

In this paper, we address refugees' agency towards recovering camel husbandry, the conditions that permitted this process to occur and come to fruition, as well as the transformations in camel husbandry that are emerging, focusing on the case of Sahrawi refugees living in camps near Tindouf, in western Algeria[b]. Historically, camels were central to the production and reproduction of Sahrawi nomadic society, providing staple food, means of transport and warfare, means of exchange and the basis of power and prestige. With war and displacement, most of the Sahrawi who fled lost their camel herds, became refugees settled in camps and depended on international food aid for survival. Although several authors reported the recovery of livestock husbandry among Sahrawi refugees at the turn of the millennium (Bhatia [2001]; Caratini [2007b]; Mundy[2007]; de Juan Canales [2010]; Herz [2013]), little attention has been given to the trajectory pastoralism took beginning with war and sedentarization in refugee camps or to Sahrawi refugees' agentic actions to recover camel husbandry. Indeed, the Sahrawi are seldom referred to in modern literature on pastoralism; for example, they are not mentioned in Homewood's ([2008]) recent book on the ecology of African pastoralist societies and are generally absent from edited books on pastoralism (Chatty [2005]; Bollig et al. [2013]). We argue that, at the beginning of the 1990s, a co-occurrence of factors (renewed access to territory, military demobilization and increased access to cash through pensions, remittances and aid) created conditions for the re-development of productive activities, trade and the emergence of an informal economy in the camps themselves. In continuity with their nomadic past, some refugees gained access to camels and resumed camel husbandry. These processes revitalized camel-associated traditional knowledge and the material and cultural bonds between refugees and their homeland (Volpato and Puri [2014]). The camel was re-appropriated as a symbol of a shared nomadic heritage and cultural identity, and camel products and associated knowledge and practices were deployed in the Polisario's and refugees' nationalistic discourse *vis-à-vis* Morocco as well as to reinforce national and ethnic unity. As discussed at the end of the paper, the fact that Morocco has also attempted to incorporate the camel into Moroccan national identity shows that there is a continuing struggle between the two parties to claim and monopolize Sahrawi nomadic heritage.

Footnote

[b]The data and information discussed in this paper are drawn from fieldwork carried out by the first author between 2006 and 2010 in the Sahrawi refugee camps and in the liberated territories of Western Sahara. Fieldwork included a survey (about camels owned, use of camels and camel products, extent to which the herd is used for market-oriented activities, camel management, distribution of camel products, personal history of camel husbandry; $n = 74$) and semi-structured interviews ($n = 36$) with refugee and nomadic camel owners, and a survey ($n = 62$) with refugees' households about camel meat and milk procurement and consumption. Data were analysed using SPSS and Excel to derive descriptive statistics. The ethical guidelines followed were those adopted by the American Anthropological Association ([1998]) and the International Society of Ethnobiology ([2006])

After presenting the current context in the 'Background' section, in this paper, we: (1) describe how the Sahrawi became refugees and lost their herds; (2) discuss the historical, social, economic, cultural and ecological processes that facilitated the recovery of camel husbandry among Sahrawi refugees; (3) characterize contemporary camel husbandry and its importance within Sahrawi refugee camps; (4) discuss the changes that occurred in camel husbandry in the process and (5) analyse the contemporary role of camels in Sahrawi cultural and political identity.

BACKGROUND

The *Sahrawi*, literally 'people from the desert', are pastoralists who traditionally inhabited coastal areas of northwestern Africa including Western Sahara, northern Mauritania and part of southwestern Algeria. The Sahrawi were essentially nomadic, pasturing camels, goats and sheep in the low-lying plains of Western Sahara and relying for food on livestock products as well as dates, sugar, cereals and legumes that were bartered for livestock in markets on the periphery of their nomadic areas (Caro Baroja [1955]). In 1975, the Moroccan army occupied Western Sahara, forcing about 70,000 Sahrawi to flee and settle in camps established in neighbouring Algeria (San Martin [2010]). A 16-year war ensued between Morocco and the Sahrawi's armed political organization, the Polisario Front (1975 to 1991). Throughout this period, the Sahrawi were excluded from most of their former Western Sahara territory by means of a wall erected by the Moroccans (known as the *berm*) that cuts through Western Sahara in a north–south direction. Today, about 165,000 Sahrawi live in four refugee camps located on the Hamada desert plateau near Tindouf in Algeria (Figures 1 and 2).

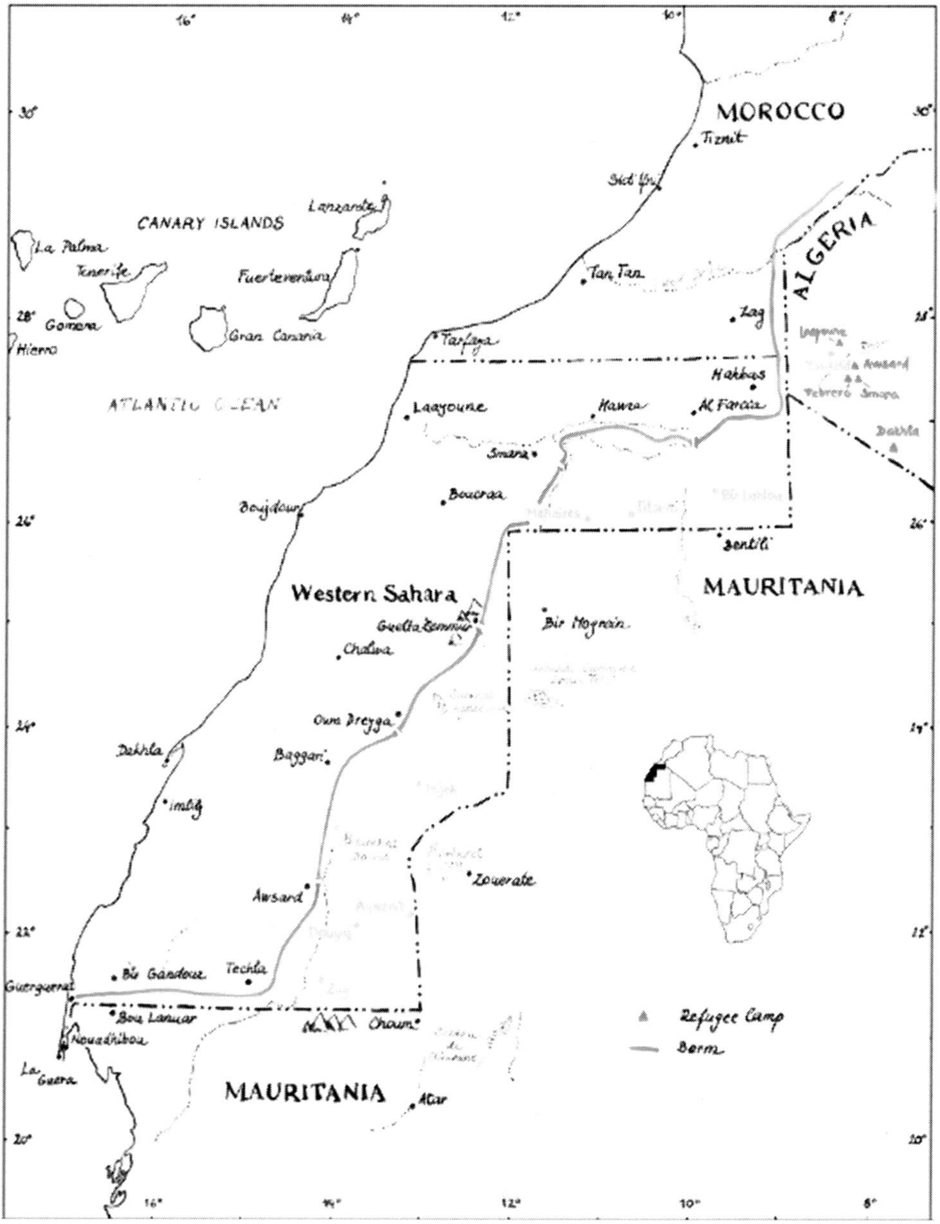

Figure 1: Map of Western Sahara with refugee camps and the liberated territories (P. Kourková).

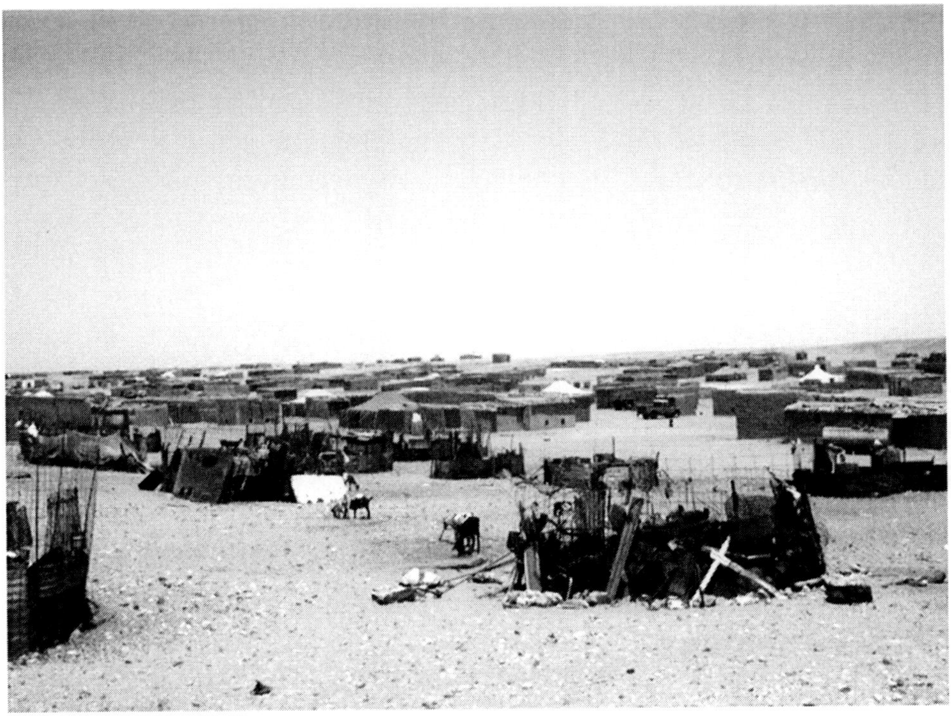

Figure 2: Sahrawi refugee camps with livestock pens in the foreground (G. Volpato).

Refugees live in tents and mud brick huts and confront continuous problems with water, food and energy supplies. Food, shelter and other basic commodities are provided by the European Union, certain bilateral development programmes, UN agencies, the Algerian government and several solidarity groups (San Martin [2010]). Over the years, refugees have attempted to improve the quality of life in the camps, developing an informal economy where they market a variety of basic consumer products as well as food. They are involved in wage labour (e.g. as butchers, mechanics, construction workers, etc.) and trade between the camps and Mali, Mauritania, Algeria and Spain (Dedenis [2005]; Herz [2013]). Some have migrated abroad and send remittances home. Economic activity has greatly increased since a United Nations-sponsored ceasefire agreement was signed with Morocco in 1991, which resulted in the demobilization of Polisario troops who moved into the camps and began to re-engage in livestock husbandry, seasonal nomadism and trade.

With the ceasefire agreement, the Polisario Front also assumed political control over the Eastern, inland areas of the Western Sahara (Bhatia [2001]), the so-called liberated territories (approximately 20% of the Western Sahara)[c] while the remaining 'occupied territories' are under the Moroccan Government's administrative authority. Pastoral areas within the liberated territories are important to the refugees' struggle to maintain or recover traditional cultural and social practices, from livestock husbandry to medicinal plant use (Volpato et al. [2012]), as well as to generate income, e.g. through the sale of desert truffles (Volpato et al. [2013b]). Some 20 to 30,000 Sahrawi who remained nomadic throughout the war by moving with their herds to safe areas in neighbouring Mauritania and Mali also reoccupied these territories after 1991, herding their livestock and using the refugee camps and Zouérat (in Mauritania) as their main commercial hubs. Today, camel husbandry is practiced in the liberated territories as well as, to a lesser extent, in the areas surrounding the refugee camps. About 2,000 camels are raised in the camps, whereas some 40,000 are raised in the liberated territories (DNV-RASD [2007]). Furthermore, the Polisario own and tend some 27,000 camels in the liberated territories, where soldiers or paid labourers act as shepherds (Broglia and Volpato [2008]). In refugee camps, camel owners supplement natural forage with fodder purchased in Tindouf. In contrast, nomads (full-time and seasonal) practice extensive camel husbandry in the liberated territories, that is, husbandry that is highly dependent on pasture areas and mobility for herd production and reproduction.

Footnote

[c]See Volpato and Rossi ([2014]) for a photographic description of the liberated territories and of local nomads' life.

Whereas, throughout their history, tribal and camp leaders (re) distributed subsistence goods and means of production in camels and organized the defense of camps, camels and territory; today, the Polisario provides and distributes aid and defends and controls the refugee camps and the liberated territories. Although refugees are highly dependent on food aid, the Polisario produces a small part of the refugees' food supply. An important part of this production comes from Polisario livestock herds[d] which directly supply refugees with fresh camel milk and she-camels loaned to disadvantaged and poorer refugees, the elderly, former combatants and their families, and gift young or male camels for slaughter, e.g. for weddings. The Polisario also allocate milk-producing camels to workers in public places such as schools and hospitals. Polisario herds also supply livestock and their products for important rituals connected with social or political events. Livestock husbandry is one of the refugees' few endogenous activities developed and recovered without any consistent attention or funding from donors and development organizations. In the past decade, camels have also been the subject of international cooperation projects promoting health and nutrition through the supply of camel milk and meat (Mundubat [2007]). These projects are carried out and funded by non-governmental organizations (NGOs) under the Polisario's initiative and largely mirror the forms of support that the Polisario provides with its herds.

Footnote

[d]In 2005, the Polisario held about 40,000 sheep, 30,000 goats and 25,000 camels (DNV-RASD[2005]).

The recovery of camel husbandry is ongoing in the refugee camps of the Hamada and in the liberated territories where refugees travel and nomads live. The Hamada is a barren desert plateau known historically as the 'Devil's Garden' because rainfall is scarce and edaphic conditions are poor, which explains why it has very poor forage resources, few trees, no halophytic plants and few annuals. Across the liberated territories, the climate is also arid and continental, with summer daytime temperatures surpassing 50°C, while winter temperatures drop to zero at night. In the territories, rain generally occurs from the end of the summer through autumn. Average annual rainfall is 30 to 50 mm; however, rains are highly irregular both within and between years, and droughts are recurrent. But, in comparison with the Hamada, the liberated territories and especially the northern area, called Zemmur, are richer in biodiversity and forage plants. After the rains, they display a savannah-like environment dominated by *Acacia* trees, and flowering prairies may appear in flat gravel areas.

WAR, SAHRAWI NOMADS AND THEIR HERDS

Morocco's occupation of the Western Sahara and the ensuing war led to the decimation of camel herds and a drastic reduction in the number of Sahrawi that remained nomadic. In 1974, on the eve of the invasion, there were some 75,000 Sahrawi, only 40% to 45% of whom were nomads (Pazzanita [2006a], [b]; Censo-74 [1974])[e] tending about 50,000 camels, as well as numerous goats and sheep (Mercer [1976b]). Prolonged droughts in the 1960s and 1970s led many Sahrawi to sedentarize in the expanding urban areas in the periphery. The number of nomads and camels had been declining in Western Sahara since at least the 1950s, but this decline assumed almost epic proportions with occupation and war and might have led to the collapse, if not of this entire population, certainly of their way of life.

Footnote

[e]This census might have missed between 7 and 10,000 nomads (Gaudio [1993], p. 61).

Although figures are far from certain, it is estimated that about 55,000 Sahrawi (or about 70% of the population) fled to the refugee camps (Mercer [1976a]), about half of whom were nomads. The Moroccan air force bombarded temporary refugee camps in Western Saharan territory (at Oum Dreiga, Mahbes, Amgala and Guelta Zemmour) with napalm, white phosphorus and cluster bombs, causing Western Sahara towns to depopulate at the same time that Tindouf refugee camps swelled (Hultman [1977])[f]. Such panic was produced among most of the Sahrawi population that they tried to escape at any cost (San Martin [2005]), leaving their homes and belongings, livestock, jobs, in many cases, ceding their moveable property (herds, jeeps and trucks) to the Polisario forces that organized and carried out both the flight and the guerrilla war that ensued to recover their territory (Lippert [1992]; Brazier [1997]). The establishment of refugee camps behind the Algerian military outpost of Tindouf in Algerian territory meant that refugees were safe from bombings and that Polisario forces had a place to train former tribesmen and organize guerrilla war (Martin [1976]).

Footnote

[f]The Moroccan Army also poisoned wells to ensure that those people and herds that were not eliminated by the bombings would be unable to occupy the territory (Lippert [1987]).

Nomads, whose resilience and herds had already been weakened and reduced by droughts and colonialism (Capot-Rey [1962]; Mercer [1976b]), had to quickly decide whether to try to maintain their herds or liquidate them and flee to safety with other refugees. Apart from the bombings and well poisonings, they risked having their herds confiscated and being forced to sedentarize, having their mobility curtailed and dealing with possible lack of pasture within and across the borders of a country engulfed in war (Arkell [1991]; Gaudio [1993]). During the war, herds were bombed, abandoned, slaughtered and sold off by different agents (Pazzanita [2006a], [b]). The Moroccan offensive against camel herds was also meant to cut off the Polisario guerrilla's food supplies and logistical support. As a consequence, the large majority of Sahrawi nomads disbanded and joined the refugee camps soon after the invasion or within the next few years. Many attempted to sell their herds before fleeing in spite of the fact that prices had plummeted and cash buyers were difficult to find. At times, fleeing nomads abandoned herds in their customary nomadic territory in the (misplaced) hope that the animals could be recovered when stability had returned. Those who managed to reach refugee camps in Algeria with their herds often had to sell them (e.g. to local Algerian nomads) cheaply because they could not be fed and managed in the camps. Probably one of the most significant phenomena within this process was the Polisario's nationalization of camel herds. Some nomads turned their herds over to the Polisario rather than attempting to sell them, and the Polisario also appropriated some of the abandoned herds[g] and sought to manage 'national' camel herds within the nomadic territories that they could access or defend. These herds supported soldiers in the field (e.g. with meat and milk, since motor vehicles rather than camels were used for transport) and at times provided fresh meat for refugees.

Footnote

[g]There are no data available about the number of camels that Polisario obtained this way.

Still, several thousand nomads did not lose their herds or flee to the camps. A report from the early 1980s (Camacho [1987]) suggests that about 10,000 Sahrawi remained nomadic by moving to safe areas (e.g. West Algeria, Mauritania, northern Mali), making use of cross-border (or transnational) social relations based on tribal membership and solidarity with the Polisario. In the new system of social relations that emerged with the war, the Polisario became a supra-tribal power able to fight for the recovery of territory, represent the Sahrawi people as a whole internationally and provide refugees with the necessary means of consumption through political and humanitarian support. Nomads provided the Polisario militia with milk and meat from camels and small livestock and in turn were protected from Moroccan incursions. Those nomads that survived slowly moved back to the liberated territories after the ceasefire agreement of 1991.

Refugees suffered tremendously from the war: when fleeing through the desert, many lost children to starvation and spouses and parents succumbed to bombings, napalm attacks and extra-judicial executions (Lippert [1992]; Hernández [2013]). Old people, women and children suffered from severe malnutrition, lack of clean water, diseases and epidemic infections (Mercer [1976a]). In this context, it was impossible for tens of thousands of sedentarized refugees to rely on their own labour and resources for survival (Wilson [2012]). Providing the population with aid in the form of food, shelter, fuel and clothing was essential (Lippert [1992]). Those first years saw a collectivist war-economy develop based on international food aid managed and delivered to refugees by the Polisario and state (Sahrawi Arab Democratic Republic (SADR)) institutions[h] which established a national administration in exile in the refugee camps (San Martin [2005], [2010]). Refugees depended on the Polisario, which assumed and transformed many of the functions played by traditional nomadic Sahrawi camps and tribes (Farah [2008]). Irrespective of previous social differences (e.g. of wealth or caste), refugees all became equal in that they lost their livelihoods and property and became dependent on aid; livestock, the former basis of wealth, were nowhere to be seen. The few refugees who managed to bring livestock to the camps had to confine them in a single public pen (Wilson [2012]), effectively collectivizing their scarce resources. As Herz ([2013]), p. 12 argued, 'much of the nomadic culture was discarded, as life in the camps did not lend itself to the keeping of large camel herds.' Private trade was prohibited in the camps, and money was not used as currency. All of this began to change with the ceasefire agreement of 1991, which led to social relaxation in the camps, with greater freedom of movement of people and goods, the emergence of a private market sector and its acceptance by Polisario authorities and new opportunities for refugees to pursue individual and family livelihood strategies. This permitted Sahrawi refugees to exercise their agency in order to recover camel husbandry, as seen below.

Footnote

[h]The SADR is a partially recognized state that claims sovereignty over the territory of Western Sahara. It was established by the Polisario Front in 1976 to provide a new entity to fill the political void left by the departing Spanish colonizers. The SADR government controls about 20% of the Western Sahara territory.

REFUGEES' RECOVERY OF CAMEL HUSBANDRY

The recovery of camel husbandry among refugees was triggered by different but interacting economic, political, ecological, cultural and social drivers. The form this took was strongly informed by the past and also strongly influenced by the nature of these drivers and of the changing context. With the material and political change stemming from the ceasefire agreement of 1991 and, given the lack of alternative livelihood pathways in the desert environment, many refugees pursued camel husbandry as a path towards food security and livelihood diversification. The ceasefire agreement granted refugees access to part of their former nomadic territory (the liberated territories) and its grazing resources. Military operations ceased and Polisario soldiers were demobilized, which meant that many men with experience in camel husbandry returned to the camps and attempted to continue their activities. Sahrawi nomads also moved back to the liberated territories with camel herds that could be sold or loaned to refugees. Now firmly under the military control of the Polisario, safety and security in the camps and the liberated territories allowed refugees to invest and travel without threat to their persons and belongings and to renew mobility by means of jeeps, which allowed them to travel to markets (e.g. Tindouf) and to their former nomadic territories. Livestock and equipment purchases were facilitated by access to cash through, among other sources, Spanish civil pensions, donations and remittances. This also stimulated the development of productive activities and trade, leading to the growth of an informal economy in the camps, as well as widespread extra-camp trade and other economic and social interactions. Refugees emigrated (e.g. to Spain) and sent remittances or repatriated earnings while establishing transnational networks through diaspora. Camel and small livestock husbandry emerged as one of the very few means to sustainably exploit the resources of the Western Sahara, facilitated by the favourable rains of the past 10 to 15 years. Camel husbandry provides refugees with their traditional staple foods - fresh milk and, to a lesser extent, meat, in a context where, as in the past, agriculture is barely possible and hunting and gathering resources are very limited. Livestock husbandry traditionally provided resources for barter and now provides access to cash. Below, this process is addressed in more detail, starting with the means by which refugees gained access to camels in the camps.

Access to Capital and the Development of an Informal Economy in Refugee Camps

Soon after Polisario soldiers were demobilized and joined refugees in the camps, they began to engage in all sorts of informal private commercial and productive activity, boosting economic life. Up to that moment, mainly women undertook the limited economic activities in the camps as they attempted to supplement consumption; former soldiers slowly refocused household activities towards production for trade and commerce. A similar transformation occurred in relation to livestock: traditionally, women managed small livestock production for own consumption and they re-initiated this during the war, whereas camel husbandry and commercial livestock production can be traced in most instances to demobilized fighters (Mundy [2007]).

A large number of refugees gained access to cash through Spanish pensions, remittances, funds obtained through the programme *Vacaciones en Paz* (Holidays in Peace), formal and informal microcredit including loans from NGOs and other refugees, and trade (de Juan

Canales [2010]; Herz [2013]). In 1988, the Spanish Government authorized pension payments to about 5,000 Sahrawi who had worked for the colonial Government of the Spanish Sahara (e.g. as public workers and troops). These pensions (400 to 500 € per month) were paid retroactively as a lump sum, so many refugees received a substantial amount, which permitted them to invest in livestock and four-wheel drive vehicles as well as provide loans or credit to others, etc. Thus, cash began to circulate in the camps and incipient commercial activity arose with Tindouf and towns in Mauritania. Since the mid-1990s, a relatively steady number of Sahrawi refugees have emigrated to work in Spain (with smaller numbers going to other countries) to support their families in the camps, and emigration was often bankrolled by Spanish pensions. Remittances (e.g. from Spain, the Canary Islands, Algeria and Mauritania) also provided ready cash. A more limited flow of remittances and other forms of assistance enters refugee camps from Sahrawi living in that part of Western Sahara that is under Moroccan administration.

Another important source of cash comes from Spanish families who host between 7,000 to 10,000 Sahrawi children per summer in Spain through a programme known as *Vacaciones en Paz*(Crivello et al. [2005], [2006]; de Juan Canales [2009]). When returning to the camps, children bring gifts for themselves (e.g. clothes, toys) and their families (e.g. solar panels, appliances and money, on average 300 € per year) provided by the host families or local solidarity associations (Morando [2006]; Crivello et al. [2006]). Some host families collect money to send to the children's families in the camps, thus greatly contributing to refugees' income and to the emergence of a cash economy (Crivello et al. [2006]). It is estimated that this injects between 500,000 € and 1,000,000 € into the camps each year (Mundy [2007]).

Since the 1990s, refugees have also benefitted from small grants and microcredit programmes offered by NGOs to initiate small enterprises (Elizondo et al. [2008]), which has boosted productive activities and self-reliance among refugees (Cavaglieri [2005]). In some cases, microcredit has directly funded camel purchases to initiate milk production (López Belloso and Mendia Azkue[2009]). Besides formal microcredit, funds are provided informally by Sahrawi refugees through credit, loans and delayed payments in market transactions, particularly to relatives and acquaintances, increasing the number of refugees with access to cash. Cash empowered refugees through forms of redistribution, as is also found with other refugee populations (Koser and Al-Ali[2001]; Horst [2006b]). On a smaller scale, refugees with no access to cash may sell part of the aid that they receive to purchase other food (e.g. fresh camel meat and milk) or non-food products (e.g. coal) (Corbet [2008]), thus allowing them to participate in the camps' market economy.

The cash entering the camps permitted petty commerce, commodity production and a market economy to develop in the camps (Shelley [2010]; Herz [2013]) involving an ever-increasing number of refugees. Together, the potential to engage in long-term investment and commercial activities, and the proliferation of informal markets both within the camps and further afield, not only provided certain pre-conditions for the resurgence of camel husbandry but as well ensured that the social and technical relations entailed in newfound pastoralism would be substantially different from the nomadic past.

The Requirements of Camel Husbandry Recovery

Sahrawi refugees have attempted to recover livestock ever since they first settled in refugee camps. It has been shown in other contexts that one strategy used to restock is to diversify economically, as income gained in other sectors can be channeled into pastoralism (Horowitz and Little [1987]). Among the Sahrawi, the recovery began with small livestock (goats and sheep) and it was only after the mid-1990s that this evolved into camel husbandry. Today, a large majority of refugee households maintain small livestock in pens around the camps (Herz [2013]); compared with camels, small livestock are more economically accessible, have higher reproduction rates and fewer nutritional requirements, are more easily sold and have a more convenient size for own consumption; hence, pastoralists commonly begin with small livestock and only upscale to camel husbandry if and when conditions permit (Dahl [1979]; Mace and Houston [1989]). During the war, refugees generally lacked means to access camels (raids were banned and refugees had insufficient capital to purchase camels) and also lacked pastures in areas surrounding the camps. Accumulating the cash to purchase a camel (about 400 to 600 €) is not easy, and camel husbandry in the camps is even more onerous since further initial investments are required for pens, water tanks and fodder, while high risks of loss are entailed due to unfavourable husbandry conditions (Broglia and Volpato [2008]). The material requirements of camel husbandry included access to camels, to fodder and pastures, to associated social networks (e.g. for labour, herd management, product distribution, etc.) and also access to the requisite camel-related knowledge.

While the recovery of camel husbandry is still rather limited in terms of the numbers of refugees and camels involved, it is highly relevant both materially and culturally. While most refugee households own some goats and sheep, very few (1% to 5%) own camels, totaling only a few thousand camels per camp. For almost all such refugees, camel husbandry is a productive activity that complements food aid and meets social and cultural expectations related to both camels and their products. Camel husbandry continues to be constrained by refugees' lack of capital and by the unfavourable environmental conditions of the camps.

Diversity of Access to Camels

With the ceasefire agreement of 1991, access to the liberated territories and the demobilization of soldiers, on the one hand, and the increased inflow of cash into the camps, on the other, began to stimulate the recovery of camel husbandry, which was further sustained by the potential to market meat and milk in the camps. Camel purchases arose, in order of importance, in the liberated territories, Mauritania, Mali, Algeria and Niger, and were sometimes embedded in elaborate trade involving the Sahrawi diaspora. A number of cases demonstrate both the fact that the strategies refugees use to access camels may be quite complex, involving a 'chain' of activities and investments, as well as the diverse motives for accessing camels. Camels are gifted and inherited, as is the case with a 15-year-old boy who received a gift of two she-camels from his father. They are also purchased from savings - a 50-year-old refugee living in the Aaiun camp initiated a commercial camel herd by purchasing camels in Mauritania with cash obtained from his Spanish pension. Some are obtained through barter: one refugee emigrated to Spain, bought two cars and then exchanged them in the camps for eight camels, which are pastured in the liberated territories using a hired shepherd and which provide milk and other use values for his family when the rains come and they move to the liberated territories to live seasonally as nomads. One refugee migrated to Spain where he worked for a year in construction and, with the money he saved, bought a second-hand truck. He travelled with the truck via boat to Nouadhibou (Mauritania), and then overland to Azawad (in northern Mali), where he exchanged the truck for about 40 camels. He then travelled back to the camps and hired shepherds to bring the camels to him. Once there, the camels were sold to local butchers for a net profit. A woman who obtained remittances from her brother working in Spain bought a milk-producing camel to provide fresh milk for her widowed father. A couple with three children bought two she-camels with money that two of the children received from their hosts in Spain. Collective agency (requiring shared aims and coordination of interdependent plans of action; Bandura [2006]) may also be involved in camel purchases usually, but not always, among kin; in at least one case, four neighbouring (non-kin) households in the camp of Aaiun purchased a milk-producing camel, sharing the costs as well as the milk produced.

Other refugees obtained camels through non-monetary social relations (e.g. from nomadic or refugee kin or acquaintances with herds) as gifts (in which camel ownership is transferred) or, more often, loans (in which ownership is not transferred and camels are used for milk production). Reciprocity involving camels and camel products was very important to the maintenance of social cohesion among Sahrawi nomads and occurred mainly through kinship in accordance with tribal organization. Contemporary redistributive mechanisms serve functions that are similar to those strategies (e.g. *mniha* - the act of lending milk-producing camels and their calves to fellow tribesmen, an institution embedded in nomadic Sahrawi society) that redistributed camel surpluses through a wider population, permitting destitute nomads to reconstitute herds or survive drought or raids. Similar institutions are present in different pastoral populations throughout the world (Faye [2009]) and, in many cases, their demise has increased pastoralist vulnerability to droughts and other stresses (McCabe [1990]) or, conversely, they have become increasingly important to the survival and functioning of these communities (Ziker [2006]).

Once Sahrawi refugees have managed to renew access to camels, these traditional institutions have been revitalized and adapted: camels and camel milk began to be redistributed through gifts and loans, permitting access to a larger refugee population. One refugee camel owner, for example, gave three 2-year-old camels as gifts, one to a family of acquaintances, another to a young man who was helping him in construction work and a third to a cousin who gave the name of the camel owner to her newborn child. These camels may be then kept for milk production or, especially if young, slaughtered to provide meat for a wedding or baptism. However, the number of refugees receiving camels as gifts is rather limited. Loans (and delayed credit) are more widespread. *Mniha* plays an important role in the re-emergence of camel husbandry among refugees, where refugee and nomadic relatives from the liberated territories, Mauritania, and even from the Moroccan-controlled territories loan the camels, or camels may be loaned within the camps, as when a 'milk project' owner (see below) loaned a she-camel to the widow of one of his former workers.

Typology of Camel Husbandry in the Refugee Camps

We have addressed how refugees managed, through economic and social means, to access camels, arguing that this access was made possible by the inflow of cash into the camps and the re-activation of social networks. Renewed access to camels, however, did not give rise to the re-emergence of traditional extensive camel husbandry among refugees, but rather led to different forms of settled or partially settled husbandry. Refugee camel pastoralists are socially differentiated, which is reflected in herd size, social-economic relations and camel management practices. Broadly, three main forms of camel husbandry can be distinguished in the camps: (1) those who produce milk for own consumption (from two to a handful of she-camels); (2) small-scale commercial milk producers (from 10 to 30 camels), who sell milk after providing for own consumption and gifts; and (3) large-scale commercially oriented meat and milk producers (30 to 100 camels). In all cases, milk and meat are sold exclusively within the camps.

Refugees in the first category keep their camels under no-grazing conditions in a pen close to the household or on the camp's periphery (Figure 3). Camels are fed food scraps, hay and fodder and are watered from wells or potable water pipes. Refugees are strongly motivated to maintain camels for milk production (Figure 4) both because it is an essential staple and marker of cultural identity and because of beliefs that camel milk has health-giving and nutritional properties, especially for the ill and the elderly. These refugees consume or give away all milk produced. Milk is gifted to relatives or neighbours or given in exchange for labour (such as for camel milking). For example, soon after receiving his Spanish pension, one 60-year-old refugee and former nomad and his family moved to the periphery of the Smara camp, built a livestock pen and bought two she-camels with their calves. Although he lost his camels after a year, he re-invested and is now very proud of his four she-camels and three calves, which provide milk for his and one of his married son's family.

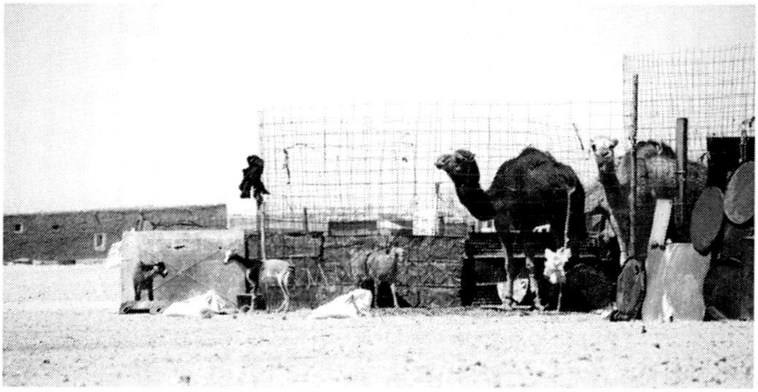

Figure 3: Camels in a pen (G. Volpato).

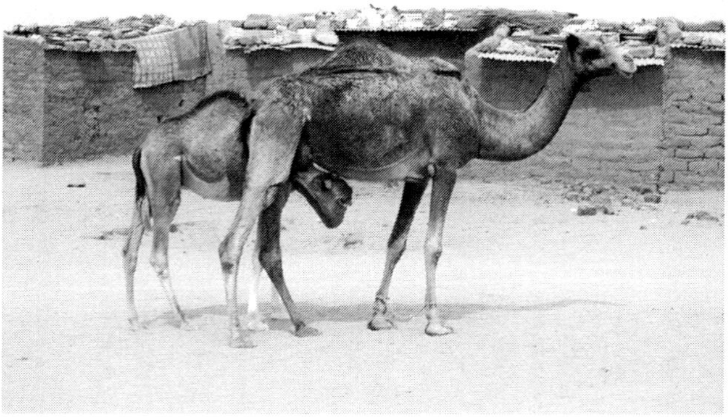

Figure 4: Camel feeding her calf in front of a refugee's house (G. Volpato).

Owners of medium-sized herds maintain most camels in free-grazing conditions in the liberated territories or in the Hamada of Tindouf, while some are kept in the camp to produce milk for own consumption, distribution and, at times, for sale. For example, one herder kept five milk-producing camels in the camp where besides providing for own consumption, a small fraction of the surplus milk produced was given away, while most was sold to cover the costs of fodder and water. This group includes many demobilized soldiers who maintain a 'traditional' approach to camel husbandry: they sell relatively small quantities of milk (e.g. 10 to 20 L per day), keeping some for themselves and for relatives and neighbours, while periodically distributing milk for free on a larger scale (some give all the milk produced on Fridays). The herd that is maintained in free-grazing conditions is usually loosely guarded if grazed around the camps or tended by nomadic relatives if grazed in the liberated territories. Such herds are used to support nomadic relatives, obtain cash from the sale of males and as a form of savings.

The third group consists of those who manage private enterprises of variable size (up to 100 camels) primarily devoted to sales of fresh camel milk (up to hundreds of litres per day) and/or meat in the camps. Their organization is more formal compared with smaller-scale producers and is based on the use of wage labour, with small quantities of milk destined for own consumption and gifted to the workforce. Milking is done by hand; milk is unpasteurized and is packaged in plastic bottles. It is taken to the camps by jeep and sold directly to refugees in local markets or indirectly via shops selling prepared food or groceries in the camps. Productive and non-productive she-camels are managed separately; milk-producing camels are kept on the periphery of the camps and fed mainly cut fodder, whereas the rest are kept under free-grazing conditions in the liberated territories or northern Mauritania. These enterprises are sometimes called 'milk production cooperatives' since some are the result of the joint investment of various refugees who then share the earnings. Milk projects have increased in number over the past decade due to increased camel milk demand. The profits obtained have generated substantial personal wealth for some. The main constraint to initiating a milk project is the lack of financial resources required to invest in a large milk herd; the funds used to date were obtained through remittances, Spanish pensions and/or earnings from other commercial activities.

Access to the Liberated Territories

The Sahrawi's traditional pastoral territory was almost inaccessible to pastoralists while engulfed in war from 1975 to 1991 but, since then, the 'liberated' areas have been key to the re-emergence of camel husbandry and camel-related practices among refugees as they provide grazing resources for refugees' and nomads' herds, as well as a place for nomads to live and refugees to move in seasonal or 'holiday' nomadism. Refugees' use of the liberated territories and northern Mauritania (where the Sahrawi have free informal access) for pasturing herds is informed by an economic rationale related to the emergent markets for livestock and livestock products in the refugee camps, as camel herds spend fallow or fattening periods in free-grazing conditions in these regions. This is especially the case for refugees with larger herds: in milk enterprises, fallow she-camels are grazed in the liberated territories as long as forage plants are available (after rains) to 'keep them healthy with good forage' and save the cost of feeding them in the camps on cut fodder. In meat enterprises, especially after rains, refugee herders use the liberated territories to fatten camels and small livestock before selling or slaughtering them in the camps.

Besides enjoying milk and meat in the camps, some refugees move seasonally with their livestock to the liberated territories where they consume these products. Some move to fatten livestock, purchasing small livestock and camels before heading for the *badiya*. One family bought about 300 goats and sheep and 40 camels which were sold upon return to the camps; in at least two cases, this system was embedded in the camel trade destined to supply meat to the camps - camels are bought in Mauritania or Mali, brought to the liberated territories where she-camels provide milk for seasonal nomadic refugees, males are fattened and, at the end of the period, sold to butchers in the camps.

Besides this economic rationale, seasonal nomadism is informed by many refugees' desire to enjoy a nomadic life in the *badiya* (Volpato and Rossi [2014]). Each autumn and/or winter, depending on the location of rains, thousands of refugees move to the *badiya* (especially its northern area) together with their livestock, tents, food stocks and various tools and other personal items, 'to graze camel herds and get away from the camps' (Mundy [2007], p. 295). Dedenis ([2005], pp. 86–87) and Caratini ([2007a], pp. 192–193) report that trips to the *badiya*may take the form of a 'holiday' (i.e. periods based on consumption rather than production), where refugees plan get-togethers with their nomadic relatives or celebrate important events (e.g. childbirths, weddings). Such seasonal nomadic strategies are encountered among other pastoral populations. In Ethiopia, for example, the refugee camps in neighbouring Somaliland were incorporated into seasonal nomadic movements so that nomads could rely on the camps' food networks during the dry season when pasture was difficult to find and milk was scarce, and refugees in turn enjoyed livestock products during the rainy season (Ryle [1992]). Boulay ([2004]) also described the phenomenon among former nomadic inhabitants of Nouakchott and other Mauritanian cities of a 'return to the *badiya*' after the rainy season for a milk and meat 'cure'.

Access to Knowledge

The knowledge a population holds about a mode of subsistence or productive activity is developed and transmitted across generations of engagement with a local environment and is commonly termed 'traditional', 'local' or 'indigenous' knowledge (Ellen et al. [2013]; Vandebroek et al.[2011]). As with other pastoral populations across the world, including the neighbouring Tuareg (Antoine-Moussiaux et al. [2007]), over the centuries, Sahrawi pastoralists have accumulated, shared and transmitted knowledge of camel husbandry in the desert environment of Western Sahara, including ethnobotanical knowledge about camel forage (Volpato and Puri [2014]), ethnoveterinary knowledge required to diagnose and treat camel diseases (Volpato et al. [2013a]) and ethnoecological knowledge about weather and rainfall patterns, soils, the location of wells and water points, distances and trajectories for transiting the desert and many other types of knowledge. With forced displacement, herd loss and sedentarization in refugee camps, knowledge transmission was disrupted. Younger people's disengagement with camels and the desert environment led to a lack of both the need and opportunities to learn. Decades of restrictions on access to nomadic territories meant there were no encounters with the learning environments in which camel and desert-related knowledge was transmitted, and knowledge acquisition and transmission became dormant (Volpato and Puri [2014]). A shift in values associated with formal education, emigration and exposure to mass media and to development schemes further alienated younger refugees from camel husbandry and the associated knowledge and cultural heritage, which some have even come to regard in negative terms.

With the resurgence of camel husbandry, which also involves young refugees who have no previous experience, many have struggled to revitalize the associated knowledge. The sources of this knowledge, principally older refugees and those who remained nomads, are involved in both vertical and horizontal knowledge transmission paths (Volpato and Puri [2014]). Recipients are not only those refugees who re-engage in camel husbandry but also political organizations and NGOs that support refugees. For the first two decades after exile, the SADR government and international organizations focused on guaranteeing the supply of basic items required for refugees' survival, and the conservation of traditional Sahrawi knowledge was not an issue of public concern. However, with the recovery of part of the Sahrawi's nomadic territory, the growing reconstitution of herds and flocks, and a string of years with favourable climatic conditions, camel-associated knowledge regained importance in the public sphere. Caratini ([2000], p. 445), for example, says that 'the Polisario Front have reconstituted a camel stock [...] and it realized that the loss of know-how in regard to livestock husbandry (based on the knowledge of the desert and of livestock needs) might represent a handicap both in the eventuality of a resumption of the war and given the perspective of peace.' In light of this, after the ceasefire agreement was signed, the Polisario involved its soldiers in a 'learning pastoral life' exercise involving nomadic shepherds (Caratini [2000]). The Polisario's revalorization of camel-related knowledge also entails the promotion of camel husbandry among younger generations and refugees as a symbol of cultural identity. For example, since 1992, the *Festival de la Cultura y de las Artes Populares* (Festival of Culture and Popular Arts) is held annually in Dakhla refugee camp, in which 'members of the older generations are actively engaged in teaching the youth a culture and traditional lifestyle that young people cannot find in school books' (SPS [2005]). Besides being crucial to camel husbandry, the recovery of camel-associated knowledge and values is functional to Polisario and Sahrawi refugees' assertions of political independence and rights to their territory as discussed below.

THE EMERGENCE OF PERI-URBAN, COMMODITIZED CAMEL HUSBANDRY

Technically and economically, the camel husbandry system developing in and around the refugee camps is quite similar to the peri-urban milk and meat camel husbandry systems that have developed around Saharan towns over the past few decades (Chaibou and Faye [2005]; Faye et al. [2003]). In fact, across arid and semi-arid areas of Africa, camel husbandry represents a viable productive pathway and has progressively become commoditized through marketing of camels and camel products in peri-urban husbandry systems. The transformation of pastoral nomads into petty commodity or capitalist producers, and of subsistence pastoral production into commodity production, has been occurring throughout Africa to various degrees and at various scales with increasing integration of camel milk and meat markets at regional and national scales (Herren[1992]; Nori et al. [2006]).

Recovery among Sahrawi refugees has thus entailed very substantial changes in environmental, technical and social relations of production and exchange compared with the nomadic past, and in several ways reflects refugees' dependence on, and engagement with, a transnational political economy. Their dependence on extra-territorial aid and income, their exposure to formal education and to formal and informal markets in the camps and abroad, their settlement in and reliance on the camps with limited access to their former territories and the fact that not all refugees are able to access the capital required to restock camel herds have all brought about such change. Below, we address three main aspects of this change, namely (1) the technological intensification of camel husbandry, (2) the commodification of camel products and (3) the establishment of new social relations around camel husbandry. We then address cultural expectations and resistance associated with these changes.

Changes in Camel Management and Technological Intensification

As the relationship with the nomadic territory disintegrated, camel husbandry in the camps came to rely far less on the biological resources of the desert and far more on imported capital and fodder. While nomadic camel husbandry depends on mobility and extensive free-grazing as main strategies to feed camel herds, refugees are sedentarized and lack grazing resources, so camel husbandry in the camps is mainly based on purchased fodder as well as flour, straw and barley grain. The economic viability of camel husbandry around the camps depends on the cost of feed and other inputs costs and access to the means to cover them. The need to purchase fodder places an economic burden on camel owners and often forces them to generate revenues from production to pay for feed; fodder is either purchased with the same sources of cash used to access camels or with revenue from milk sales.

The intensification of camel production among refugees does not occur through breeding or the use of tools or machines to substitute human labour (and thus reduce the costs of production). Rather, intensification, as understood here and as described for peri-urban camel systems in other parts of the world (Faye et al. [2003]), refers to the substitution of extensive land use (grazing on wild forage plants) with intensive input use - essentially, camels are confined in a smaller spaces and live from purchased fodder, trucked in water supplies and modern veterinary medicines. Different authors have noted a more general tendency in Saharan camel husbandry towards reduced mobility and grazing intake and increased consumption of fodder and supplementary feeds (Michel et al. [1997]; Faye et al. [2003]). Throughout the last century or so, the use of supplementary livestock feeds has increased worldwide in part as a result of the increasing availability of cheap agro-industrial by-products and mechanized transport systems capable of delivering them in bulk (Blench [2001]).

In most cases, fodder is purchased in Tindouf. Travel and trade, including for fodder purchase, are facilitated by the diffusion of vehicle transport that, since the 1990s, greatly facilitated refugees' mobility (Dedenis [2005]). After the war, jeeps and trucks have superseded camels as a means of transport. Camels now provide transport only on a limited scale and only among nomads, but few nomadic households regularly move to new grazing areas with their belongings packed on camels. Although, as Bulliet ([1975]) described so brilliantly, for 2,000 years, the camel managed to displace the wheel in North Africa and the Middle East, in the 20th century, the wheel, now coupled with the internal combustion engine, took its revenge, and the use of camels for transport went into steep decline. The widespread use of jeeps and trucks in desert environments has had profound impacts on camel pastoralists' lifestyle (Chatty [1980], [1986]). Owning a 'land rover' is a principle ambition among Sahrawi refugees and one of the first commodities they acquire when they have sufficient cash is a motor vehicle. These facilitate trade and inter-camp transit, serving as taxis and transporting goods to and from Tindouf, the liberated territories and Mauritania. People ride camels in the camps only during SADR political or ritual celebrations when mounted camel parades are performed to demonstrate the Sahrawi's nomadic origins (Figure 5). The camel has become a symbol of Sahrawi cultural identity in public and political rituals and demonstrations as, for example, in 1997, when James Baker, the former UN mediator of the Polisario-Morocco conflict, visited the camps and again in 2006, in Tifariti, for the 30th anniversary of the SADR's foundation.

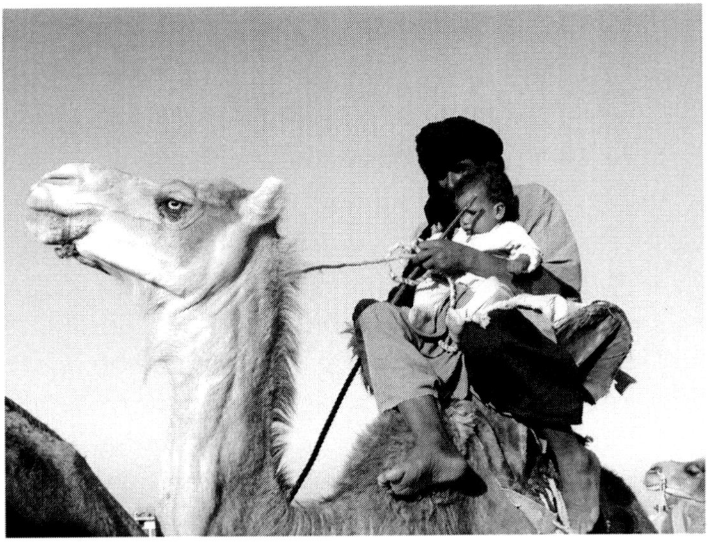

Figure 5: Camel riding during a political celebration in Rabouni refugee camp (G. Volpato).

The diffusion of motor vehicles has also changed camel management. Most successful refugee camel owners own a jeep or truck. Especially market-oriented camel herders use other complementary technologies such as tanker trucks, GPS and satellite phones. Trucks make it easier to supplement camels' diets with harvested wild plants, hay and fodder. The historical constraints related to water provision for camels are addressed by developing new wells, mechanization (pumps) and tanker trucks that bring water to the herds, which obviates the need to move herds to water. There is generally increased reliance on owned or rented tanker trucks both among refugees and nomadic herders, particularly for larger, market-oriented herds. Herds can exploit grazing resources in the liberated territories that would otherwise be too distant from water points, whereas in the camps, it permits large herds to be maintained on the periphery where water is deposited in large tanks.

Camel Milk Commodification

Although historically, the Sahrawi traded surplus camels, an unprecedented process of commodification of camels and camel products is occurring among refugees. Camels are no longer bartered for food and other essentials but are sold for profit; meat is sold in butcher shops and milk, which it was formerly taboo to sell, is subject to widespread trade and high consumer demand. As trade gave rise to an informal economy in the camps, camel milk has become at least partly commoditized, as have other natural products that were previously not subject to monetary exchange, such as plant medicines and desert truffles (Volpato et al. [2013b]).

Studies investigating Sahrawi refugees' dietary intake confirm that camel milk is widely consumed (Henjum et al. [2010]; Grewal [2011]). Refugees source camel milk in three ways: (1) own production, which is very limited due to the small number of refugees who own or maintain camels; (2) social mechanisms of redistribution in which refugee camel owners, the Polisario Front and certain international NGOs maintain milk-producing camels in and around the camps and provide refugees with fresh milk through family, social and/or political networks; and (3) purchase in camp shops and directly from refugee producers, which accounts for the majority of the milk consumed in the camps. About half of the refugee camel owners surveyed by the first author ($n = 44$) sell camel milk. Nomads ($n = 30$), however, do not sell camel milk but rather, as in the past, redistribute it through kinship and other networks, to neighbouring households that have no milk-producing camels and to labourers that manage herds as well as to their families.

The commodification of camel milk in Sahrawi refugee camps reflects trends reported in urban markets across Saharan Africa (Faye et al. [2003]), from the Western Sahara under Moroccan administration (Michel et al. [1997]) and Mauritania (Abeiderrahmane [2005]) to Kenya (Noor et al.[2013]) and Somalia (Farah et al. [2007]); the same trends are found, for example, in Saudi Arabia (Faye et al. [2014]). Commodification occurs through two possible paths: through the penetration of capitalist relations of production, and/or as a necessary adaptation to husbandry in sedentary conditions. The second particularly applies to Sahrawi refugees; camels had to be fed purchased fodder. Sahrawi refugees were forced to incorporate fixed and variable capital to substitute resources otherwise obtained for free in their traditional territories. In order to obtain the capital needed to maintain camels in the camps, refugees began to sell at least part of their milk. In a few but far-reaching cases, this led some refugees to develop large herds and seek profits. At the same time, these changes have been met with resistance on the part of some refugees with a nomadic background who challenge changes that have occurred such as the commodification of camel milk, which has fundamentally altered social relations and challenged traditional values and beliefs. Indeed, the Sahrawi have maintained a more traditional approach in nomadic conditions (e.g. in the liberated territories), where the redistribution of camel milk still constitutes the basis of the nomadic community, giving credibility to the idea that it is need, rather than greed, that has led to milk commodification.

Social Relations around Camel Husbandry

Over the past 50 years, Sahrawi social relations and political organization have undergone no less than a revolution. Major social and political change commenced with colonialism and war and culminated with exile and the creation of a Sahrawi nation-state, the SADR (see footnote h). Historically, the Sahrawi were organized politically in tribes, where several inhabited the traditional territories (e.g. Reguibat, Izarguien, Oulad Delim, Oulad Tidrarin, etc.; see Briggs

[1960]; Pazzanita [2006a], [b]) in a segmentary system that further subdivided each tribe into branches based on extended families and other kinship ties (Hart [1998]; Caro Baroja [1955]). Tribal relations determined access to pasture where each tribe controlled a customary nomadic area. Decision-making institutions and networks of mutual support functioned along tribal lines and especially within branches (Caratini [1989]). The tribes of Western Sahara continuously interacted through trade, war, raids, agreements of mutual access to each other's customary areas (e.g. with drought), alliances, tribute payments, etc. Although this political organization was disrupted with colonialism, it was in the mid-1970s that it was completely overturned by events: with exile and the establishment of the camps, the Polisario banned tribes and reorganized the Sahrawi under a newly declared nation-state in which each refugee became a citizen of the SADR and pledged allegiance to the Polisario, which controls and grants refugees access to the liberated territories and manages food aid (Wilson [2012]; Caratini [2003]). While kinship continues to have considerable importance among contemporary Sahrawi, tribal affiliation gave way to Polisario allegiance, and the Polisario Front de facto assumed the functions previously assumed by tribes and extended this to incorporate other functions of the modern nation-state, e.g. international political representation. Among Sahrawi refugees, social relations have been established and/or reformulated around camel husbandry on the basis of kinship (e.g. between refugees and nomads) and on Polisario governance (e.g. for access to the liberated territories).

The process transforming tribal authority to a nation-state is exemplified by the changes that occurred in camel brands. Branding refers to cauterizing unique symbols (marks) on an animals' body to communicate information about ownership, the owner's social status and grazing rights (Landais [2001]; Humphrey [1974]). Brands are also essential elements of identity in pastoral societies, as their collective character serves as an assertion of collective rights (e.g. of tribes) to specific resources (e.g. water, pastures) (Landais [2001]; Bernus [1996]). Among Sahrawi nomads, the process of branding camels was known as *mhar* (*nar* in Arabic) or *elama*; camels were usually branded on the neck or the thigh, or on the head or other visible part of the body (Caro Baroja [1955]; Boyer [1962]). Each tribe had its own brand, while larger tribes (e.g. the Reguibat in the 19th century) had different brands for major segmentary branches. Monteil ([1952]) recorded more than 25 brands used by Sahrawi tribes or their bands, about half of which incorporated letters or combinations of letters from the Arabic alphabet (e.g. the letters *kaf* and*qaf* for the Reguibat), the rest consisting of stylizations or abstract symbols.

The origins of brands were usually embedded in myths that tied into a single narrative the tribe's founder, the camel and the brand (Caro Baroja [1955], pp. 89–90). Camel brands conveyed the power of a tribe not only in terms of the number of camels held but also the location of camel herds in the territory - an indicator of territorial control. The brand, then, was a message conveyed to other pastoral groups about the related priority of access (or not) to the territory where those camels grazed. Thus, for pastoralists, the brand can be considered as a functional and symbolic equivalent of national flags for claiming territorial occupation and defining which human groups are granted access.

In the social revolution from a tribal to a state organization led by the Polisario, brands were also revolutionized. Today, all camels belonging to Polisario are marked on the neck with the letters 'FP' (Frente Polisario) followed by a number relating to a military region (from one to seven). For Polisario herds, this brand has completely displaced tribal marks, including a noticeable shift in the alphabet from Arabic to Latin, and a shift in the symbolic function of these herds' identity, from one based on tribal divisions to one based on Sahrawi unity. The Polisario adopted the branding conventions of the colonial authorities - Spanish and French colonial powers branded their herds with numbers rather than symbols. Polisario brands thus represent a rejection of traditional tribal symbols, reinforcing the ideological unity of the Sahrawi people beyond tribes and draw upon colonial symbols of state ownership. However, in continuity with the tribal past, in the liberated territories, the presence of camels marked with 'FP' indicates control over those territories and its resources and hence to whom people owe allegiance when using those resources.

With the recovery of camel husbandry and renewed access to a shared nomadic territory, refugees began to interact more intensively with nomads, often on the basis of kinship ties. Some nomads and their herds became integrated with the camel-based economy emerging in the refugee camps by functioning as reservoirs of camels (e.g. through loans) and camel-related knowledge and as a source of camel milk for refugees engaging in seasonal nomadism. Nomads in turn use the refugee camps as a commercial hub where they sell livestock, procure other items, access aid through refugee relatives and exchange food with refugees. As Wilson ([2012]) also noted, both refugees and nomads use the liberated territories to graze herds, interacting in a vast network of solidarity and reciprocity that is strengthened by kinship ties linking nomadic and refugee households. The common interest in camel husbandry has largely defined their relationships, served to strengthen social bonds that were severed with the dissolution of tribes and contributed to the development of a system of apparent mutual benefit.

The Sahrawi case is not the first in which refugee camps are shown to have a positive impact on regional economies by functioning as commercial hubs for local nomads who sell their surplus animals in the camps. Jansen ([2011]) reports the same for the Kakuma camps of Kenya. There, however, nomads and refugees are from different and rather antagonistic ethnic groups; the former are Turkana and the latter mainly Dinka, so that the relations between them are strictly based on trade. Among the Sahrawi, there is a deep interpenetration between refugees and nomads, so that patterns of exchange involve extended families and reciprocity, in addition to market exchange.

In the past, labour relations around camel husbandry were based on extended families and on structural differences within and between tribes. While poorer nomads relied on own and male kin labour, more powerful nomads and tribes (i.e. with hundreds of camels) exploited the labour of slaves and dispossessed nomads (e.g. members of a defeated tribe) (Caro Baroja [1955]; Hart[1962]). Today, nomads and refugees with small non-commercial herds still rely principally on family labour. However, in market-oriented enterprises, labour relations around camel husbandry have been largely commoditized, representing a break from the types of structural social differences that prevailed in the past. Commercially oriented herders use hired labour for camel management (e.g. feeding and watering) in and around the camps and contract shepherds to tend herds in the liberated territories. In the camps, labour is mainly provided by young refugees who have little formal education. In the liberated territories, refugee youth, Sahrawi nomads (local or from Mauritania) or, in some cases, sub-Saharan migrants are contracted. Shepherds are paid in cash rather than in kind whereas, in the past, they were paid in livestock, e.g. a camel in exchange for a year's labour.

Cultural Expectations and Resistance around Camel Husbandry

Refugees do not share the same attitudes towards the recovery of camel husbandry and renewed access to camel products, nor to the changes in camel husbandry and camel management. The refugee literature identifies two contrasting processes of cultural change in situations of exile (Couldrey and Morris [1999]; Volpato and Waldstein [2014]). The first is a tendency towards loss or abandonment of traditional culture, which is maintained only among elderly and specific, often marginal, groups. The second is a process of maintenance or recovery of traditional culture in order to promote the maintenance or recovery of productive activities and cultural identity. Among Sahrawi refugees, those who have been at least partly acculturated in the West and many other younger refugees who have never experienced nomadic life often express less concern about cultural continuity and regard camels and camel husbandry as 'backward' unless they are used as a means to make money. Older and more culturally conservative refugees stress the importance of livestock and livestock products, especially camel milk, and demand that their children meet their expectations by consuming camel milk and meat and travelling to the liberated territories.

Incentives to recover camel husbandry include the desire, especially of older refugees, to consume fresh camel milk and spend at least part of their lives in the *badiya*. Dedenis ([2005]) writes that sons continue to be motivated by the social obligation to provide fresh livestock products for their parents and to reconstitute herds; feelings of good health, pride, dignity and freedom are associated with a 'return to the *badiya*'. For the elderly, travelling through space to the *badiya* represents travel in time back to their youths. The *badiya* and its key elements (green deserts after rains, livestock, camel milk, tents) are emblematic of the culture they represent - of nomadic Sahrawi - and of associated values such as freedom and autonomy[i].

Footnote

[i]An association between 'freedom' and the '*badiya*' is often found in nomadic Sahrawi poetry, which was largely based on the description and celebration of *badiya* resources and landscapes. For example, the most renowned living Sahrawi poet, Mohamed Mustafa Salem (known as Badi) said, 'In the *badiya*a man is free to do everything he pleases, with his life, with his livestock, with his water. He is owner of himself. Who does not live in the *badiya* cannot be owner of himself, in any other place...Every minute of life one feels free, very free. Nothing is better in the *badiya* than when a friend comes, a person you esteem and to whom you can offer everything you can imagine' (cited in Gimeno Martín and Pozuelo[2010], pp. 11–12) [own translation from Spanish].

Forms of cultural resistance arose among refugees around technological change and intensification, where some are against the use of tanker trucks to water camels, which 'corrupts nomadic life'. Because traditional camel pastoralists have internalized camels' needs and the constraints of camel husbandry into their systems of knowledge and beliefs about the natural world, in their eyes, such change goes against the laws of nature. Some believe that, although tanker truck water comes from wells, it is not as good for camel's health as water that is directly extracted from wells and that camels watered directly with well water have greater strength and stamina[j]. Similarly, some traditional herders are 'against fodder' and are proud of the fact that they rely exclusively on free-grazing resources, believing that purchased fodder is bad for camels' health and lowers their resistance. The dialectic between 'innovation' and 'tradition' in camel management has, in some cases, assumed the form of an intergenerational struggle in which older men tend to favour traditional strategies. These forms of cultural resistance are probably an integral part of situations where profound change in the mode of subsistence and social relations are underway and have also been shown to occur among Sahrawi refugees in relation to concepts of illness, health and healing (Volpato and Waldstein [2014]).

Footnote

[j]According to Elmi ([1989]), Ceeldheer pastoralists of Somalia do not like to water their camels from wells with a motorized pump for two reasons: the camels do not like the water because it smells of diesel, and water stored in metal tanks is cooler than that from the bottom of the well, and thus, camels do not like it and will not drink it to capacity.

THE CAMEL AND SAHRAWI IDENTITY

All the people like us are we, and everyone else is they (Rudyard Kipling, We and They, 1926).

Kohler-Rollefson ([1996], p. 283), in her work on the origin, use and dispersal of the one-humped camel in Asia, writes, 'The function of animals in human societies is usually not restricted to utilitarian purposes; they often fulfil important and culturally distinct symbolic and ritual roles...and quite frequently develop into hallmarks of identity.' Historically, among the Sahrawi, the camel was not only the material pillar of society but as well the cornerstone of Sahrawi tribal and nomadic identity. Several Sahrawi tribes' origin myths were based on camels (Caro Baroja [1955]; Mercer[1976a]); camels were central to Sahrawi beliefs, sayings and poems (Pinto Cebrián [1997]); camel ownership defined prestige and social rank; and nomads identified with and felt affection for their camels and their local camel breeds. With recovery, much of the cultural significance of the camel as a symbol of ethnic identity has been revitalized, which is reinforced by the Polisario's efforts to create and sustain a national identity based on ethnicity, cultural heritage and territorial occupation.

Identity refers to feelings of belonging to a specific group based on a distinctive shared language, culture, social organization and ideology (Hurskainen [1990]; Snow [2001]). Identities and their symbols are continuously constructed and re-constructed by redefining the differences between the self and the other, the cultural borders in which these differences are represented, and abandoning or adopting different key elements of identity (Drzewiecka [2002]; Nagel [1994]). As Corbet ([2008]) noted, contemporary Sahrawi are struggling in multiple ways to reconstruct their identity. The camel is a central, figurative and symbolic element that represents the Sahrawi and differentiates them from other (non-camel pastoralist) populations. The re-establishment of a relation with the *badiya* based on pastoral and nomadic practices reaffirms Sahrawi refugees' cultural identity based on their nomadic origins.

When the Polisario overturned tribal social structure, it eliminated the basis of social differences in favour of national unity, social equality and Sahrawi collective identity and citizenship and, at the same time, the cultural and political significance of camels was undermined. This revolution was necessarily cultural as well as social; tribalism in all its forms, as well as the material basis of this tribalism, were antithetical to the Polisario's project of building the basis for nationalist claims to the territory against other nationalist claims (e.g. Morocco). The Polisario thus not only eliminated (prohibiting reference to) tribal institutions and affiliations but as well discouraged the transmission of tribal myths of origin, which affirmed the distinct genealogical identities of the Sahrawi tribes as well as the symbolic significance of the camel as the material and cultural basis of these tribes' existence. As the Polisario nationalized camel herds, the camel was purged of any significance as the basis of tribal or personal power in favour of a cultural identity based on the unity of all ethnic Sahrawi under a 'modern' nation-state. However, the camel was too potent a symbol both of Sahrawi ethnic identity and of Sahrawi claims to their traditional nomadic territory to discard wholly or permanently. The camel was later to be recovered as a symbol of Sahrawi unity *vis-à-vis*other populations and so regained a prominent place in Sahrawi cultural identity not only among refugees and nomads engaged in camel husbandry but as well in official Polisario discourse and practices. For the Polisario, the rebirth of the camel's symbolic significance was functional to claims of independence. Camel husbandry reinforces the Polisario's claims to nation-statehood by legitimizing control over the former territory pertaining to the Sahrawi nomadic tribes both through occupation (people and animals) and use and by providing for the national welfare and reducing dependence on foreign aid by means of state food production and redistribution. The camel and camel husbandry also serve to legitimize claims to national identity by representing the basis of a shared ethnic, cultural and political identity, as well as symbolizing the differences between the Sahrawi and other populations, particularly the Moroccans.

The contrasting political ideologies and claims of the Polisario, on the one hand, and of the Morocco Government, on the other hand, constitute a crucial axis of the dispute over control of Western Saharan territory. Under the Polisario, Sahrawi identity has been reinforced on the basis of differences between the Sahrawi and the Moroccans, whose cultural practices are explicitly and implicitly contrasted (Chamberlain [2005]). The SADR's Ministry of Information produces educational and informational material for refugees that stress this contrast in terms of language, food, dress and women's roles (Allan [2010]) and, as a result, 'many aspects of everyday Saharawi existence become cultural markers' (Chamberlain [2005], p. 27). This is also the case with ethnobotanical knowledge associated with the desert environment and camel husbandry (Volpato and Puri [2014]), which contrasts with Morocco's agricultural traditions. The dispute over Western Sahara territory thus aims to 'hegemonise a collective social imaginary about what it is to be Saharawi, who the Sahrawis are and who the 'others' are that delineate the frontier of 'our Sahara' (San Martin [2005], p. 587). Camels and camel husbandry are part of this dispute and are central to the public representation of Sahrawi political identity. Camels appear in refugees' and Polisario's discourses as the basis of a 'stolen' nomadic life in the *badiya*, where 'pastures are good' and 'camels gain health', in contraposition to neighbouring areas (e.g. Morocco to the north, central Mauritania to the south) where 'camel diseases are widespread' and 'the climate is too wet for camels'. Below, we present three examples of this re-appropriation of the camel as a symbol of cultural and national identity in relation to the figure of the *deyar* (a nomad who searches for stray camels), to the skills needed to slaughter camels and to the use of camel milk in political contexts.

In Sahrawi nomadic culture, the *deyar* is a very knowledgeable and experienced nomad camel tracker who locates camels that have strayed in the desert and returns them to their herds. *Deyars*read tracks in the sand and infer a great amount of information from their shape, depth, distribution, direction, etc. *Deyars* are highly respected for their knowledge, skills and intimate relation with the desert environment. With the collapse of nomadism during the war and the changes that ensued in camel management (e.g. increased reliance on motor vehicles and binoculars), the number of *deyars* drastically declined and their skills are being lost. But if their physical presence is dwindling, their cultural significance is not: on the contrary, *deyars* have a prominent place in present-day Sahrawi literature and poetry (see for example Ebnu [2008]; Boicha et al. [2003]; Bahia [2007]; Moure [2004]), where they often represent the *badiya* itself and the lost relationship with and knowledge of Western Sahara territory. At the same time, the*deyar*'s search for stray camels has come to symbolically represent the Sahrawi's search for the camels lost with the war and, in a wider sense, of the search for their lost nomadic life, independence, and freedom in the territory of Western Sahara, and hence an assertion of the claim to the territory.

Among the cultural practices that the Sahrawi contrast explicitly with the Moroccans are camel slaughter skills, which reflect the intimate relation between camels and the Sahrawi as well as the alleged Moroccan's ignorance of camels. The contrast is stressed by a young Sahrawi author who describes a camel slaughterhouse on the outskirts of El Aaiún city in Moroccan-controlled Western Sahara, where camels can be heard crying out in suffering, which he contrasts with Sahrawi practices known as *nosh* (Autores Varios [2009], pp. 89–90)[k]. One of the *nosh* prescriptions dictates that, when slaughtering a camel, suffering must be minimal, which is possible only through the skills and experience of the slaughterer, which are transmitted between herders across generations as part of Sahrawi cultural heritage. So, for example, when a young Sahrawi attended an encounter with King Hassan II in 1979 organized by the Moroccan authorities, they sacrificed a camel: it 'was horrible, that animal was crying a lot… those people don't have any idea of how a camel must be killed' (A.A. [1979]). Indeed, if the main arteries between the neck and the thorax are severed with a single cut, death occurs instantaneously, whereas if the cut is not expertly executed, death is delayed and the animal suffers (Farah and Fischer [2004]). In pre-colonial Sahrawi society, usually, the eldest or most respected man slaughtered camels, which was forbidden to lower social groups (e.g. slaves). Thus, a contraposition that was internal to the social system (slaves-camel owners) has been conceptually reorganized as an external contraposition (Moroccans-Sahrawi), which is functional to Polisario political struggles and claims to Sahrawi unity.

Footnte

[k]*Nosh* literally refers to tethering camels by grabbing them by the tail.

Since at least 1999, the struggle for Sahrawi nationhood has extended into that part of Western Sahara under Moroccan control where the Sahrawi experience social and economic discrimination and participate in nationalistic demonstrations and riots (San Martin [2005]). In this context, camels are an issue; a group of former nomads from El Aaiún is currently campaigning for compensation for the camel herds that Moroccan troops killed during the war, which requires the Moroccan authorities' recognition that troops were ordered to butcher Sahrawi herds, a fact that Moroccan authorities deny (Shelley [2004]). Such acts are contrasted with the Sahrawi's affection for the animal and the social and the cultural importance attached to camels and camel products. Sahrawi who struggle for independence in the Moroccan-controlled Western Sahara adopt camel milk as a symbol of their ethnic and national identity while reflecting the difference with Moroccans' sedentary lifestyles and identities. Reports show that, in April 2006, when Moroccan authorities released Sahrawi activists from prison and again in Agadir, in 2007, when Sahrawi students were released for having publically demanded independence for Western Sahara, their Sahrawi supporters greeted them with cups of camel milk and dates (SPS [2006], [2007]), just as Sahrawi nomads returning from long desert treks were received in their camps in pre-colonial times.

Morocco is also promoting camel husbandry in the part of Western Sahara under its control while attempting to appropriate the camel as a symbol at a sub-national (i.e. ethnic, tribal) level, thus proposing that Sahrawi nomadic heritage is part of Moroccan national heritage (Martin-Márquez[2006]; Julien [2004]). Polisario calls for Sahrawi unity *against* tribal identity, while Morocco tries to promote and enhance tribal identity and downplay or deny the existence of Sahrawi national unity (Corbet [2008]). Moroccan authorities are attempting to undermine the Polisario's monopoly over the politicization of Sahrawi nomadic culture, exalting the camel and its characteristics. This has occurred in the context of a parallel recovery of camel husbandry in Moroccan-controlled Western Sahara which has been on-going since the 1990s, especially with the emergence of commercial enterprises producing and selling camel milk and meat (Pazzanita [2006a], [b]; Michel et al. [1997]). The Moroccan Government and local authorities increasingly fund camel husbandry, supporting it through direct aid (e.g. subsidies for camel purchases), cooperation programmes that distribute free veterinary medicines and vaccines and implement applied research (e.g. epidemiological studies) (El Abrak [2000]; Essemlali [2008]; Michel et al. [1997]). Today, the Moroccan Government and media portray camel husbandry as an integral part of the Moroccan economy and promote the camel milk and meat consumption (El-Katab [2008]). Among other events promoting camel meat and milk in Western Sahara, the Moroccan authorities organized an International 'Salons of the Dromedary' in 2008 and 2009 in what they call the 'Southern Provinces' or 'Moroccan Sahara' to celebrate 'the central symbol of the culture and life of Saharan inhabitants', as the francophone Moroccan newspaper *Le Matin du Sahara et du Maghreb*(Essemlali [2008]) reported: a clear example of the attempt to reposition Sahrawi nomadic heritage as part of Moroccan heritage. Thus, a struggle to ideologically appropriate Sahrawi nomadic cultural heritage continues between Moroccan authorities and the Polisario, with the former aiming to incorporate it as a specific ethnic/tribal heritage *within* Moroccan national culture and the latter aiming to recover nomadic cultural heritage as the foundation of Sahrawi independence and against Moroccan claims[I].

Footnote

[I]See Wallerstein ([1987]) for a discussion of the political manipulation of concepts of identity as 'national', 'ethnic' or 'racial' where 'peoplehood' is 'in no sense a primordial stable social reality, but a complex clay-like historical product of the capitalist world economy through which the antagonistic forces struggle with each other' (p. 85), which seems entirely appropriate in the context of Western Sahara.

CONCLUSIONS

This study has addressed the material and cultural importance of camels and camel husbandry among Sahrawi refugees, as well as their efforts to recover their territory and productive activities and promote their shared nomadic heritage and cultural identity. The case illustrates both how refugees struggle to recover their livelihoods in contexts of forced displacement and sedentarization in refugee camps and how this struggle is informed by pre-exile modes of subsistence and cultural values. The camel was central to Sahrawi nomadic society both materially and culturally. With war and forced displacement, the Sahrawi lost most of their camels - it took decades for refugees to recover camel husbandry by regaining access to camels, grazing territory and camel-associated knowledge and to establish reciprocal relations around camel husbandry in the liberated territories with remaining nomads. Although this recovery is sustained by traditional values and practices related, for example, to camel milk consumption and redistribution, fundamental changes have also occurred: the camel lost its traditional functions as a means of transport, warfare and non-monetary exchange; management has intensified with the use of fossil fuels and motor vehicles and increasing reliance on purchased fodder and other inputs rather than on desert grazing resources; and camel products as well as access to camels and labour have been largely commoditized. The camel has also been appropriated as a symbol of Sahrawi cultural identity both by refugees and in Polisario discourse and practice, which asserts the Sahrawi's nomadic cultural heritage as a key element of a national identity legitimating claims to nationhood and traditional territories for the Sahrawi people.

The findings of this study are significant for understanding both refugees' individual and collective agency towards cultural and economic recovery and dispossessed pastoralists' struggle to rebuild herds and livestock-based forms of livelihood. We have expanded our knowledge of Sahrawi refugees' agency and their re-engagement with pastoralism and the liberated territories and also provided a framework for more generally conceptualizing some of the processes by which refugees living in camps engage in productive activities, how these are informed by their culture, access to means of production and financial capital and how they are embedded within larger-scale socio-economic change processes including commodification and migration. The findings also contribute to the understanding of human-nature relations in contexts of forced displacement and of the means by which refugees re-engage with traditional productive activities, knowledge and environmental relations, in the process adapting (and reinventing) the past to new conditions and values arising from their experience as refugees. Knowledge of these processes is important not only to understand refugees' and displaced people's struggles but also to comprehend broader cultural and social processes taking place in refugee camps (and, within this, the role of food aid) and to formulate ways in which the international community can address refugees' problems within these processes. NGOs working in refugee camps can use studies about the recovery of refugees' livelihoods to identify and implement means to assist this recovery.

Although the recovery of camel husbandry is rather limited in terms of the numbers of refugees and camels involved, it is likely to continue into the future as refugees continue to break the chains of food dependency, as long as it can be sustained by rains, and as long as access to camels and to the liberated territories remain assured. The strategy that refugees pursue leads towards greater integration of refugee camps with wider economic and social networks, but this depends on the continued existence of the camps and of international aid. As long as this trend continues, there will be an increasing number of camels and greater integration between refugees and nomads (often within extended families), creating a single productive network between the refugee camps and the liberated territories. If the referendum for Sahrawi self-determination is eventually held[m] and refugees move back to Western Sahara, some refugees might return to nomadism, merging with nomads on both side of the berm and using Western Sahara towns as commercial hubs. In this scenario, the Polisario Front might redistribute its camels to refugees, in a sort of concluding cycle in which the herds that the Polisario acquired from disbanding nomads at the beginning of the war and used to support refugees in the decades of exile, once again become the basis for a return to desert nomadic pastoralism.

Footnote

[m]The ceasefire agreement of 1991 included a referendum for self-determination originally scheduled for 1992, in which the Sahrawi would have the option to decide between independence and integration with Morocco. However, this referendum was never held and is still in the UN's to-do list (Pazzanita [2006a], [b]).

AUTHORS' CONTRIBUTIONS

GV designed the methods approach, carried out field work, analysed the data, composed the literature review and drafted the manuscript. PH participated in the study design, in the literature review and in drafting the manuscript, as well as editing it. Both authors read and approved the final manuscript.

ACKNOWLEDGEMENTS

We are very grateful to many Sahrawi for the patience, kindness and hospitality that they showed during fieldwork. We thank the Italian NGO Africa 70 - especially Alessandro Broglia, Sara Di Lello and Davide Rossi - and the Veterinary Service of the SADR (Sahrawi Arab Democratic Republic) and its director Saleh Mohamed Lamin for logistical support and cooperation. Our gratitude also extends to the Polisario personnel who accompanied Gabriele Volpato in his travels across the liberated territories of Western Sahara. Funds were granted to Gabriele Volpato by Ceres Research School of Wageningen University, The Netherlands, as part of his PhD research on the subsistence practices and ethnobiological knowledge of Sahrawi refugees.

REFERENCES

1. 1979. La extraña aventura de Chefid Mohamed. El Pais, Madrid.
2. Abbas, B, AA Al-Qarawi, and A Al-Hawas. 2002. The ethnoveterinary knowledge and practice of traditional healers in Qassim Region, Saudi Arabia. Journal of Arid Environments 50: 367–379.
3. Abeiderrahmane, N. 2005. Modern Dairy Products from Traditional Camel Herding: An Experience in Mauritania. In Desertification Combat and Food Safety, Series I: Life and Behavioural Sciences, vol. 362, ed. Faye B, Esenov P, IOS, Amsterdam.
4. Adano, WR, and K Witsenburg. 2005. Once Nomads Settle: Assessing Process, Motives and Welfare Changes on Marsabit Mountain. In As Pastoralists Settle: Social, Health, and Economic Consequence in Marsabit District Kenya, ed. Fratkin E, Roth EA, 105–136. Kluwer Academic/Plenum, New York and London.
5. Allan, J. 2010. Imagining Saharawi women: the question of gender in POLISARIO discourse. The Journal of North African Studies 15 (2): 189–202.
6. 1998. Code of Ethics of the American Anthropological Association.
7. Antoine-Moussiaux, N, B Faye, and GF Vias. 2007. Tuareg ethnoveterinary treatments of camel diseases in Agadez area (Niger). Tropical Animal Health and Production 39: 83–89.

8. Arkell, T. 1991. The decline of pastoral nomadism in the Western Sahara. Geography 76 (331): 162–166.
9. Bahia, MA. 2007. Versos Refugiados. Poesía Saharaui Contemporanea. Universidad de Alcala, Alcala de Henares.
10. Bandura, A. 2006. Toward a psychology of human agency. Perspectives on Psychological Science 1 (2): 164–180.
11. Bernus, E. 1996. Marques de propriété touarègues et pierres tombales (plaines au sud-ouest de l'Aïr). Sahara 8: 7–18.
12. Bhatia, M. 2001. The Western Sahara under Polisario control. Review of African Political Economy 28: 291–298.
13. Blench, R. 2001. 'You can't go Home again': Pastoralism in the new Millennium. Overseas Development Institute, London.
14. Boicha, L, L Lehsan, S Ebnu, S Abdalahi, AS Iselmu, and C Mahmud. 2003. Bubisher. Poesía Saharaui Contemporánea. Puentepalo, Las Palmas de Gran Canaria.
15. Bollig, M, M Schnegg, and H Wotzka. 2013. Pastoralism in Africa: Past, Present and Future. Berghahn, Oxford.
16. Boneh, D. 1984. Returning to pastoralism: three cases from the Negev Bedouin. Nomadic Peoples 15: 41–50.
17. Boulay, S. 2004. Quand un Objet Change de Statut: Trajectoire de la Tente Dans la Société Maure (Mauritanie). Ethnographiques.org 6, .
18. Boyer, JR. 1962. Contribution à l'étude de l'élevage Camelin au Sahara Occidental. Le Regueibat et son Chameau. Ecole Nationale Veterinaire D'Alfort, Paris.
19. [http://www.newint.org/features/1997/12/05/light/] Brazier, C. 1997. Light in the Darkness. : New Internationalist magazine (297).
20. Briggs, LC. 1960. Tribes of the Sahara. Harvard University Press, Cambridge.
21. Broglia, A, and G Volpato. 2008. Pastoralism and displacement: Strategies and limitations in livestock raising by Sahrawi refugees after thirty years of exile. Journal of Agriculture and Environment for International Development 102 (1/2): 105–122.
22. Bulliet, R. 1975. The Camel and the Wheel. Harvard University Press, Cambridge.

23. Camacho, A. 1987. Pastores en la guerra. El Pais, Madrid.
24. Capot-Rey, R. 1962. The Present State of Nomadism in the Sahara. The Problems of the Arid Zone. UNESCO, Paris.
25. Caratini, S. 1989. Les Rgaybat (1610–1934). 2: Territoire et Société. L'Harmattan, Paris.
26. Caratini, S. 2000. Système de parenté Sahraoui. L'impact de la révolution L'Homme 154–155: 431–456.
27. Caratini, S. 2003. La Republique des Sables: Anthropologie d'une Revolution. Editions Harmattan, Paris.
28. Caratini, S. 2007. La prison du temps. Les mutations sociales à l'oeuvre dans les camps de réfugiés sahraouis Deuxième partie: l'impasse Afrique contemporaine 2 (222): 181–197.
29. Caratini, S. 2007. La prison du temps. Les mutations sociales à l'oeuvre dans les camps de réfugiés sahraouis. Première partie: la voie de la révolution. Afrique contemporaine 1 (221): 153–172.
30. Caro Baroja, J. 1955. Estudios Saharianos. Consejo Superior de Investigaciones Cientificas, Madrid.
31. Catley, A. 2006. Use of participatory epidemiology to compare the clinical veterinary knowledge of pastoralists and veterinarians in East Africa. Tropical Animal Health and Production 38: 171–184.
32. Cavaglieri, S. 2005. Livelihood Strategies and Food Security in Refugee Camps. University of Roma Tre, Rome.
33. 1974. Censo, ed. Censo y Estadistica Servicio de Registro de Poblacion. Servicio de registro de poblacion, censo y estadistica, El-Ayoun.
34. Chaibou, M, and B Faye. 2005. Fonctionnement des élevages camelins de la zone périurbaine d'Agadez au Niger: enquête typologique. Revue d'Élevage et de Médecine Vétérinaire des Pays Tropicaux 58 (4): 273–283.
35. Chamberlain, R. 2005. Stories of a Nation: Historical Narratives and Visions of the Future in Sahrawi Refugee Camps. Refugee Studies Centre, University of Oxford, Oxford.
36. Chatty, D. 1980. The Pastoral Family and the Truck. In When Nomads Settle: Processes of Sedentarization as Adaptation and Response, ed. Salzman P, 80–94. Praeger, New York.

37. Chatty, D. 1986. From Camel to Truck: The Bedouin in the Modern World. Vantage, New York.
38. Chatty, D. 2005. Nomadic societies in the Middle East and North Africa: Entering the 21st century. In Handbook of oriental studies. Section 1 The Near and Middle East. Brill, Leiden.
39. Corbet, A. 2008. Nés Dans les Camps. Changements Identitaires de la Nouvelle Génération de Réfugiés Sahraouis et Transformation des Camps. École des Hautes Études en Sciences Sociales, Paris.
40. Couldrey, M, and T Morris. 1999. Culture in Exile. Forced Migration Review. The Refugee Studies Centre in association with the Norwegian Refugee Council/Global IDP Project, Oxford.
41. Crivello, G, E Fiddian, and D Chatty. 2005. The transnationalisation of care: Sahrawi refugee children in a Spanish host program. Refugee Studies Centre, Oxford.
42. Crivello, G, E Fiddian, and D Chatty. 2006. Holidays in peace: Sahrawi children visit Spain. FMR 25: 59–60.
43. Dahl, G. 1979. Suffering Grass: Subsistence and Society of Waso Borana. Stockholm Studies in Social Anthropology. University of Stockholm, Stockholm.
44. de Juan Canales, D. 2009. Imaginación y reacción en los Campamentos de refugiados saharauis: construcción de la cotidianeidad e identidad frente al otro extranjer (nasrani) en el contexto de la diáspora. Perifèria - Revista de recerca i formació en antropologia 10: 1–24.
45. de Juan Canales, D. 2010. Emergencia civil y economía del refugio en los campamentos de refugiados saharauis de Argelia. Gazeta de Antropologia 26 (1): 11.
46. Dedenis, J. 2005. La Mobilité Régionale de la Société Sahraouie des Camps de Réfugiés. Une Ressource Pour un Mieux-Vivre?. Université de Poitiers, Poitiers.
47. DNV-RASD. 2005. Census 2005. República Árabe Democrática Sahrawi, Rabuni, Polisario refugee camps: Dirección Nacional de Veterinaria, Ministerio de Salud Pública Sahrawi, RASD.
48. DNV-RASD. 2007. Census 2007. República Árabe Democrática Sahrawi, Rabuni, Polisario refugee camps: Dirección Nacional de Veterinaria, Ministerio de Salud Pública Sahrawi, RASD.

49. Drzewiecka, JA. 2002. Reinventing and contesting identities in constitutive discourses: between Diaspora and its others. Communication Quarterly 50 (1): 1–23.

50. Ebnu, A. 2008. Nómadas en el Exilio. Asociación Cultural Almenara, Marbella.

51. El Abrak, A. 2000. Encadrement Sanitaire du Cheptel Camelin au Maroc. In Maladies Parasitaires et Infectieuses du Dromadaire, ed. Dakkak A, 9–14. Actes Editions, Rabat.

52. Elizondo, L, CM Mehdi, and M Sanz. 2008. Microcréditos en el Sáhara. Manual Para la Solicitud de Crédito en los Campamentos Saharauis. Hegoa, Bilbao.

53. El-Katab, A. 2008. La viande du dromadaire, un produt sahraoui jusque-lá inexploité. Libération, Rabat.

54. Ellen, R, SJ Lycett, and SE Johns. 2013. Understanding Cultural Transmission in Anthropology: A Critical Synthesis. Berghahn Books, Oxford.

55. Elmi, AA. 1989. Camel Husbandry and Management by Ceeldheer Pastoralists in Central Somalia. Botany and Range Science Department, Faculty of Agriculture, Somali National University, Mogadishu.

56. Essemlali, M. 2008. Provinces du Sud: Le dromadaire symbole central dans la culture sahraouie. Le Matin, Rabat.

57. Farah, R. 2008. Refugee camps in the Palestinian and Sahrawi national liberation movements: A comparative perspective. Journal of Palestinian Studies 38 (2): 76–93.

58. Farah, Z, and A Fischer. 2004. Milk and Meat from the Camel: Handbook of Products and Processing. vdf Hochschulverlag AG, Zurich.

59. Farah, Z, M Mollet, M Younan, and R Dahir. 2007. Camel dairy in Somalia: limiting factors and development potential. Livestock Science 110: 187–191.

60. Faye, B. 2009. Pauvreté et Solidarité Chez les Peuples Pastoraux. In L'élevage, Richesse des Pauvres, ed. Duteurtre GB, Faye B, 77–87. QUAE, Versailles.

61. Faye, B, M Bengoumi, and A Barkat. 2003. Le Développement des Systémes Camélins Laitiers Périurbains en Afrique. In Lait de Chamelle Pour l'Afrique, 115–125. Niamey: Atelier sur la Filière

Laitiére Caméline en Afrique Niamey, 5–8 November, 2003. FAO Production et Santé Animales, Niamey.

62. Faye, B, H Madani, and AH El-Rouili. 2014. Camel milk value chain in Northern Saudi Arabia. Emir J Food Agric 26 (4): 359–365.
63. Fiddian-Qasmiyeh, E. 2011. The pragmatics of performance: Putting 'faith' in aid in the Sahrawi refugee camps. Journal of Refugee Studies 24 (3): 533–547.
64. Gaudio, A. 1993. Les Populations du Sahara Occidental. Editions Karthala. Paris:
65. Gauthier-Pilters, H. 1961. Observations sur l'ecologie du dromedaire dans le Sahara Nord-Occidental. Mammalia 25 (2): 195–280.
66. Gertel, J, and R Le Heron. 2011. Economic Spaces of Pastoral Production and Commodity Systems: Markets and Livelihoods. Ashgate, Farnham.
67. Gimeno Martín, JC, and LM Pozuelo. 2010. Memorias orales en el Sáhara Occidental: la poesía en hasanía. 7th Congress of African Studies. Lisboa 21: 1–27.
68. Golooba-Mutebi, F, and SM Tollman. 2004. Survival to livelihood strategies for Mozambican refugees in South Africa. FMR 20: 28–29.
69. Grewal, NK. 2011. Iodine Status and Thyroid Function Among Lactating Women in Saharawi Refugee Camps, Algeria. Akershus University College, Akershus.
70. Hart, DM. 1962. The social structure of the Rgībāt Bedouins of the Western Sahara. Middle East Journal 16 (4): 515–527.
71. Hart, DM. 1998. The Rgaybat: Camel nomads of the Western Sahara. The Journal of North African Studies 3 (4): 28–54.
72. Harvey, P, and J Lind. 2005. Dependency and Humanitarian Relief: A Critical Analysis. Humanitarian Policy Group, Overseas Development Institute, London.
73. Henjum, S, I Barikmo, AK Gjerlaug, AM Lehabib, A Oshaug, TA Strand, and LE Torheim. 2010. Endemic goitre and excessive iodine in urine and drinking water among Saharawi refugee children. Public Health Nutrition 13 (9): 1472–1477.

74. [http://www.elmundo.es/elmundo/2013/10/20/internacional/1382244113.html] Hernández, R. 2013. La Semilla de la Verdad. : Sáhara Documental. . Accessed 20 Oct 2013.

75. Herren, UJ. 1992. Cash from camel milk: the impact of commercial camel milk sales on garre and gaaljacel camel pastoralism in southern Somalia. Nomadic Peoples 30: 97–113.

76. Herz, M. 2013. From Camp to City: Refugee Camps of the Western Sahara. ETH Studio Basel, Lars Müller, Zürich.

77. Homewood, K. 2008. Ecology of African pastoralist societies. James Currey Ltd., Oxford.

78. Horowitz, MM, and P Little. 1987. African Pastoralism and Poverty: Some Implications for Drought and Famine. In Drought and Hunger in Africa: Denying Famine a Future, ed. Glantz M, Cambridge University Press, Cambridge.

79. Horst, C. 2006. Refugee livelihoods: Continuity and transformations. Refugee Survey Quarterly 25 (2): 6–22.

80. Horst, C. 2006. Transnational Nomads. How Somalis Cope With Refugee Life in the Dadaab Camps of Kenya. Studies in Forced Migration. Berghahn Books, New York.

81. Hultman, T. 1977. The struggle for Western Sahara. Issue: A Journal of Opinion 7 (1): 27–32.

82. Humphrey, C. 1974. Horse brands of the Mongolians: a system of signs in a nomadic culture. American Anthropologist 1: 471–488.

83. Hurskainen, A. 1990. Levels of identity and national integrity: the viewpoints of the pastoral Maasai and Parakuyo. Nomadic Peoples 25–27: 79–92.

84. 2006. ISE Code of Ethics (with 2008 additions).

85. Jacobsen, K. 2002. Livelihoods in conflict: the pursuit of livelihoods by refugees and the impact on the human security of host communities. International Migration 40 (5): 95–123.

86. Jacobsen, K. 2005. The Economic Life of Refugees. Kumarian, Bloomfield.

87. Jansen, BJ. 2011. The Accidental City: Violence, Economy and Humanitarianism in Kakuma Refugee Camp, Kenya. Wageningen University, Wageningen.

88. Julien, Z. 2004. L'identité Sahraouie en Questions. In L'Ouest Saharien, ed. Abjean A, Julien Z, 131–231. L'Harmattan, Paris.
89. Keenan, J. 2003. The last nomads. Nomadism amongst the Tuareg of Ahaggar (Algerian Sahara). Journal of North African Studies 8 (3–4): 163–192.
90. Khalif, ZK, and G Oba. 2013. Gaafa dhaabaa - the period of stop': Narrating impacts of shifta insurgency on pastoral economy in northern Kenya, c. 1963 to 2007. Pastoralism: Research, Policy and Practice 3: 1–14.
91. Kohler-Rollefson, I. 1996. The one-Humped Camel in Asia: Origin, Utilization and Mechanisms of Dispersal. In The Origins and Spread of Agriculture and Pastoralism in Eurasia, ed. Harris DR, 282–292. UCL, London.
92. Köhler-Rollefson, I. 2003. A treatise on life with camels. German Research 1: 15–19.
93. Koser, K, and N Al-Ali. 2001. New Approaches to Migration? Transnational Communities and the Transformation of Home. Routledge, London.
94. Landais, E. 2001. The marking of livestock in traditional pastoral societies. Revue scientifique et technique de l'Office international des épizooties 20 (2): 445–462.
95. Lentz, E, CB Barrett, and J Hoddinott. 2005. Food aid and dependency: implications for emergency food security assessments. IFPRI Discussion Paper 12(2).
96. Lippert, A. 1987. The human costs of War in Western Sahara. Africa Today 34 (3): 47–59.
97. Lippert, A. 1992. Sahrawi women in the liberation struggle of the Sahrawi people. Signs 17 (3): 636–651.
98. López Belloso, M, and I Mendia Azkue. 2009. Local human development in contexts of permanent crisis: Women's experiences in the Western Sahara. Journal of Disaster Risk Studies 2 (3): 159–176.
99. Mace, RH, and AI Houston. 1989. Pastoralist strategies for survival in unpredictable environments: a model of herd composition which maximises household viability. Agricultural Systems 30.
100. Martin, P. 1976. Tribesmen swell Polisario ranks. The Times, London.

101. Martin-Márquez, S. 2006. Brothers and others: fraternal rhetoric and the negotiation of Spanish and Saharawi identity. Journal of Spanish Cultural Studies 7 (3): 241–258.

102. McCabe, J. 1987. Drought and recovery: livestock dynamics among the Ngisonyoka Turkana of Kenya. Human Ecology 15 (4): 371–390.

103. McCabe, J. 1990. Success and failure: the breakdown of traditional drought coping institutions among the pastoral Turkana of Kenya. Journal of Asian and African Studies 25 (3–4): 146–160.

104. Mercer, J. 1976. The cycle of invasion and unification in the Western Sahara. African Affairs 75 (301): 498–510.

105. Mercer, J. 1976. Spanish Sahara. G. Allen, London.

106. Meyer, S. 2006. The 'refugee aid and development' approach in Uganda: Empowerment and self-reliance of refugees in practice. New Issues in Refugee Research. Research Paper 131. :Geneva.

107. Mezhoud, S, and C Oxby. 2013. Disentangling 'Forced displacement' from Pastoral Mobility: Recovery and Reconstruction in the Sahel and in South Sudan. In Modern Pastoralism and Conservation: Old Problems, new Challenges, ed. T Sternberg and D Chatty, 210. The White Horse, Cambridge.

108. Michel, JF, M Bengoumi, P Bonnet, K Hidane, K Zro, and B Faye. 1997. Typologie des systèmes de production camelins dans la province de Laâyoune, Maroc. Revue d'Élevage et de Médecine Vétérinaire des Pays Tropicaux 50 (4): 313–323.

109. Mohamed, HA, and AN Hussein. 1996. Pastoralists: their knowledge untapped. Journal of Camel Practice and Research 3: 143–145.

110. Monteil, V. 1952. Essai sur le Chameau au Sahrara Occidental. Etudes Mauritaniennes. Centre IFAN - Mauritanie, Saint-Louis du Senegal.

111. Morando, M. 2006. La Diaspora Saharawi in Italia. Universitá degli Studi di Bologna, Bologna.

112. Moure, G. 2004. La Zancada del Deyar. El Cobre, Barcelona.

113. Mundubat,. 2007. Acta de la II Mesa de Coordinación y Concertación. In Mesa de Concertación de Soberanía Alimentaria del Sahara. Madrid :.

114. Mundy, JA. 2007. Performing the nation, pre-figuring the state: the Western Saharan refugees, thirty years later. Journal of Modern African Studies 45 (2): 275–297.

115. Nagel, J. 1994. Constructing ethnicity: creating and recreating ethnic identity and culture. Social Problems 41 (1): 152–176.

116. Noor, IM, AY Guliye, M Tariq, and BO Bebe. 2013. Assessment of camel and camel milk marketing practices in an emerging peri-urban production system in Isiolo County, Kenya. Pastoralism: Research, Policy and Practice 3(28).

117. Nori, M, MB Kenyanjui, MA Yusuf, and FH Mohammed. 2006. Milking drylands: the marketing of camel milk in North-east Somalia. Nomadic Peoples 10 (1): 9–28.

118. Pazzanita, AG. 2006. Western Sahara: anatomy of a stalemate. International Journal of African Historical Studies 39 (1): 151–154.

119. Pazzanita, AG. 2006. Historical Dictionary of Western Sahara. Historical Dictionaries of Africa. The Scarecrow, Oxford.

120. Pinto Cebrián, F. 1997. Proverbios Saharauis. Miraguano Ediciones, Madrid.

121. Ryle, J. 1992. Notes on the repatration of Somali refugees in Ethiopia. Disasters 16 (2): 160–168.

122. Salzman, PC. 1980. When Nomads Settle: Processes of Sedentarization as Adaptation and Response. Praeger, New York.

123. San Martin, P. 2005. Nationalism, identity and citizenship in the Western Sahara. The Journal of North African Studies 10 (3): 565–592.

124. San Martin, P. 2010. Western Sahara: The Refugee Nation. University of Wales Press, Cardiff.

125. Shelley, T. 2004. Endgame in Western Sahara: What Future for Africa's Last Colony?. Zed Books, London.

126. [http://www.redpepper.org.uk/sons-of-the-clouds/] Shelley, T. 2010. Sons of the Clouds. Accessed 2 Sept 2011.

127. Snow, DA. 2001. Collective Identity and Expressive Forms. In International Encyclopedia of the Social and Behavioral Sciences, ed. Smelser NJ, Baltes PB, 2212–2219. Elsevier Science, Oxford.

128. SPS. 2005. Segunda Jornada del Festival: Inauguración del Mukkayem Tradicional. Rabouni, Tindouf, Algeria. Accessed 29 Apr 2006.
129. 2006. Recibimiento Triunfal a Tamek en Assa. Assa: Sahara Press Service, Rabouni, Tindouf, Algeria.
130. 2007. Acogida Triunfal a los Estudiantes Saharauis en la Universidad Ibn Zohr de Agadir (Marruecos). Sahara Press Service, Agadir.
131. Vandebroek, I, V Reyes-García, UP Albuquerque, R Bussmann, and A Pieroni. 2011. Local knowledge: Who cares? Journal of Ethnobiology and Ethnomedicine 7(35).
132. Varios, A. 2009. La Fuente de Saguia. Relatos de a Generación de la Amistad Saharaui. Imprenta Provincial de Zaragoza, Zaragoza.
133. Volpato, G, and R Puri. 2014. Dormancy and Revitalization: The Fate of Ethnobotanical Knowledge of Camel Forage among Sahrawi Nomads and Refugees of Western Sahara. Ethnobotany Research & Applications, Accepted.
134. [http://www.smashwords.com/books/view/433218], Volpato, G, and D Rossi. 2014. Badiya: Los Nómadas Saharauis del Sáhara Occidental, ed. Smashwords.
135. Volpato, G, and A Waldstein. 2014. Eghindi among Sahrawi refugees of Western Sahara. Med Anthropol: Cross-Cultural Studies in Health and Illness 33 (2): 160–177.
136. Volpato, G, P Kourková, and V Zelený. 2012. Healing war wounds and perfuming exile: the use of vegetal, animal, and mineral products for perfumes, cosmetics, and skin healing among Sahrawi refugees of Western Sahara. Journal of Ethnobiology and Ethnomedicine 8 (49): 1–19.
137. Volpato, G, A Di Nardo, D Rossi, SM Lamin Saleh, and A Broglia. 2013a. 'Everybody knows', but the rest of the world: the case of a caterpillar-borne reproductive loss syndrome in dromedary camels observed by Sahrawi pastoralists of Western Sahara. Journal of Ethnobiology and Ethnomedicine 9(5).
138. Volpato, G, D Rossi, and D Dentoni. 2013. A reward for patience and suffering - Ethnomycology and commodification of desert

truffles among Sahrawi refugees and nomads of Western Sahara. Economic Botany 67 (2): 147–160.

139. Wallerstein, I. 1987. The construction of peoplehood: racism, nationalism, ethnicity. Sociological Forum 2 (2): 373–388.

140. Wilson, A. 2012. Households and the production of public and private domains: revolutionary changes in Western Sahara's liberation movement. Paideuma 58: 19–43.

141. Ziker, JP. 2006. The social movement of meat in Taimyr, Northern Russia. Nomadic Peoples 10 (2): 105–122.

Chapter 2

Animal Viruses, Bacteria, and Cancer: A Brief Commentary

Jimmy T. Efird[1], tephen W. Davies[2], Wesley T. O'Neal[3], and Ethan J. Anderson[4]

[1]Department of Public Health, Brody School of Medicine, East Carolina University, Greenville, NC, USA

[2]Department of General Surgery, University of Virginia School of Medicine, Charlottesville, VA, USA

[3]Department of Internal Medicine, Wake Forest University School of Medicine, Winston-Salem, NC, USA

[4]Department of Pharmacology and Toxicology, Brody School of Medicine, East Carolina University, Greenville, NC, USA

ABSTRACT

Animal viruses and bacteria are ubiquitous in the environment. However, little is known about their mode of transmission and etiologic role in human cancers, especially among high-risk groups (e.g., farmers, veterinarians, poultry plant workers, pet owners, and infants). Many factors may affect the survival, transmissibility, and carcinogenicity of these agents, depending on the animal-host environment, hygiene practices, climate, travel, herd immunity, and cultural differences in food consumption and preparation. Seasonal variations in immune function also may increase host susceptibility at certain times of the year. The lack of objective measures, inconsistent study designs, and sources of epidemiologic bias (e.g., residual confounding, recall bias, and non-randomized patient selection) are some of the factors that complicate a clear understanding of this subject.

INTRODUCTION

Humans and animals have coexisted since the beginning of time, sharing viruses, bacteria, and perhaps the etiology of cancers. Approximately 75% of viruses and 50% of bacteria known to cause disease in humans are zoonotic and can be transmitted between animals and people (1). While evolution has provided adaptive immunity against microbes and cancer, the ability to defend against infection is sometimes absent or compromised. Excluding ionizing radiation, sunlight, and tobacco, infection represents the main known cause of human cancers throughout the world. The list is long including cancers of the anogenital track (HPV), stomach (*H. pylori*), liver (HBV, HCV, liver flukes), bladder (schistosoma hematobium), prostate (XMRV), and other specific cancers such as adult T-cell leukemia (HTLV-1), Kaposi sarcoma (HHV-8), Merkel Cell Carcinoma (MCPyV), and Burkitt's lymphoma (EBV) (2, 3). The prevalence and persistence of tumor viruses varies in different parts of the world. Nearly 30% of cancers in developing and tropical countries are attributable to infectious causes compared with 10% in developed countries (4). However, the connection between viruses, bacteria, and cancer, and the role of animals, remains unclear or paradoxical in nature.

VIRUSES

An infectious etiology for cancer was first documented in animals during the early part of the nineteenth century with the diagnosis of pulmonary adenocarcinoma in sheep (later attributable to jaagsiekte sheep retrovirus) (5). Animals are the host species for many oncogenes. Among the most studied are rodent (Abl, Int1/Wnt1, Int2, Notch1, Pim1/2, Runx, Tpl2), fowl (Erb-b, Fos, Myc, Src), feline (Myc), and fish (cyc) (6). For example, reticuloendothesliosis virus readily induces cancer in chickens (avian leucosis/sarcoma). The virus has been found in eggs intended for human consumption and vaccines prepared in eggs (7). A wide variety of viruses, mirroring their human analogs, are ubiquitous among animals in nature and their habitat (e.g., fecal coliform contamination) (8–10). Common types include viruses in the polyoma, adeno, retro, and papilloma family.

Animal viruses potentially express oncoproteins in human cells even though stringent replicate restrictions exist in the latter (11). The "hit and run" hypothesis posits that certain viruses interfere with the hosts immune system to cause cancer, yet do not integrate into the victims DNA (leaving no detectable fingerprints) (12). Newborn hamsters infected with polyoma virus have been shown to develop cancers, even though the cells of this species do not support virus replication (13). Similarly, tumors induced in immunocompetent mammals with Rous sarcoma virus do not present neutralizing antibodies (14). In contrast, some animal viruses [e.g., feline leukemia virus (FeLV)] have been observed to replicate *in vitro* in human cells (15, 16). Sera collected from 69% of 107 persons among 46 households with at least 1 FeLV gs-a positive cat tested positive for antibodies against FeLV (15). Although it is unclear exactly how antibodies directed toward animal viruses could have oncogenic or mitogenic effects on host cells, these findings support the idea that long-lasting "biological memory" of animal virus exposure can exist within the host in the absence of direct effects on host DNA.

BACTERIA

Animal bacteria also have been implicated in cancer. The occurrence of gliomas in the brain of fowl have been noted in several reports (17–19) and these tumors have been described as having the pathognemonic encephalitic features of a pleomorphic parasite infection (e.g., hypertrophy and hyperplasia of blood-vessels; perivascular infiltration by lymphocytes, plasma cells, and monocytes; and the presence of A-D bodies) (20). Chickens spontaneously and experimentally infected with toxoplasma have been observed to develop glioma-like tumors (21, 22). A study of 16 human brain tumors observed bodies indistinguishable from the C and D phases of the fowl parasite (23). Epizootic outbreaks of toxoplasmosis have been reported in various avian species and mammals (22,24, 25). Furthermore, toxoplasma antibodies have been isolated in the blood of exposed sheep farmers, flock animals, herder dogs, mice, and rats (26). Potential cellular mechanisms by which animal viruses and bacteria lead to tumorgenesis are shown in Figure 1.

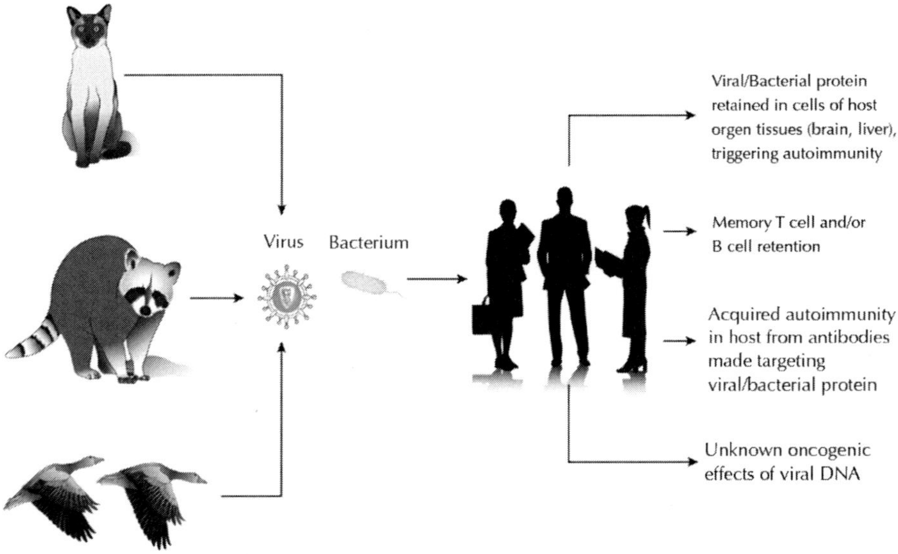

Figure 1: Potential mechanisms of carcinogenic "biologic memory" retained from exposure to animal viruses and bacteria.

AGE OF EXPOSURE

Early age at first exposure is critical for the development of many malignancies (27). Fetal or early childhood exposure to infectious agents occurs at a vulnerable time when the immune system is less developed and possibly more susceptible to tumor formation (28). The unrecognized persistence of an oncovirus or microbe in the host increases the chance for this agent to alter the cell cycle and immortalize cells (2, 29). Inoculation of immunologic immature neonate mice with polyoma virus results in tumor formation at multiple sites. In contrast, older mice do not develop tumors in response to polyoma virus either in the laboratory or by natural infection (13). The selective sensitivity of the fetus is further demonstrated in a study of patas monkeys wherein the administration of known carcinogenic agents in the fetal stage cause more tumors than an equivalent dose administered to juvenile monkeys (27, 30). Furthermore, few tumors developed when treatment was delayed until the start of the second trimester, suggesting that sensitivity was greatest during the first trimester.

TRANSMISSION

Exposure Routes and Factors Influencing Transmission

Human exposure may occur in many ways – preparing and consuming animal products, washing with, and drinking well water contaminated with animal fecal coliform, animal bites/scratches, and working in occupations involving regular contact with animals, manure, soil, and/or by-products (e.g., farmers, slaughtering plant workers). Even living down-wind of a farm field fertilized with animal manure poses a potential risk. A list of major sources and exposure routes of animal-to-people transmission of viruses and bacteria is shown in Figure 2. Factors influencing the probability of disease transmission involve the proximity and temporal contact with the infectious organism, length of time that the infectious agent is present, virulence of the agent, incubation period, stability of the agent under varying environmental conditions, population density of carrier animals, husbandry practices, and control of wild rodents and insects (31). The type and maintenance of animal housing also may affect the extent to which individuals working in or around such facilities are exposure to zoonotic viruses and bacteria. Often, animal containment structures (e.g., hen houses, pig pens, cattle barns, and horse stables) may be inadequately ventilated and/or have poor waste removal systems, increasing the exposure of animals and their caretakers to dust, fecal matter, and microbes (32).

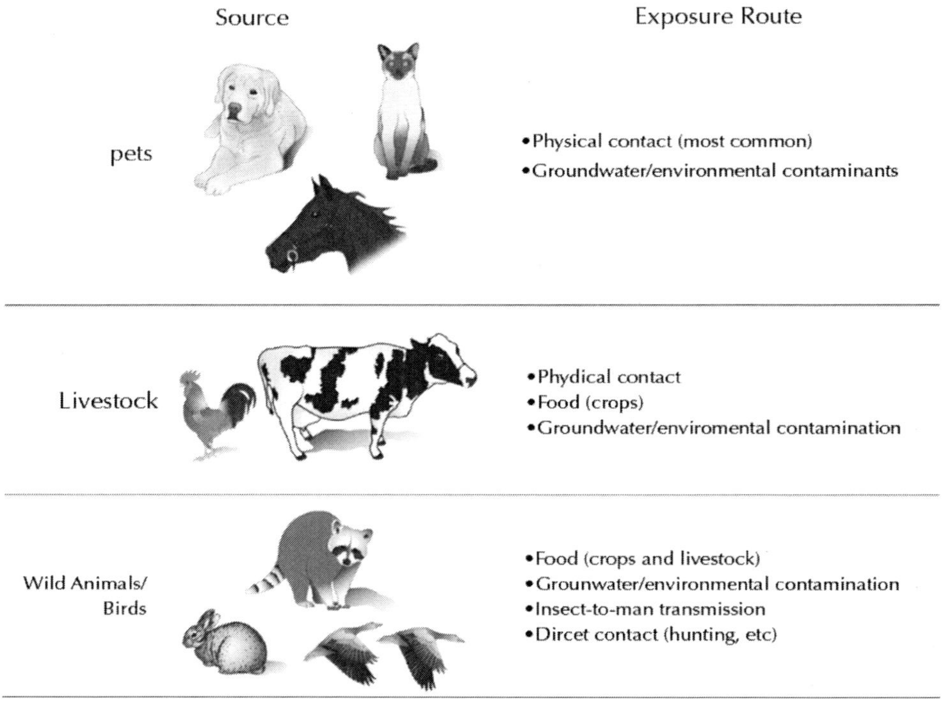

Figure 2: Routes of transmission and human exposure to animal viruses and bacteria.

Mechanical Intermediate Hosts

Infectious agents may be transmitted to humans by direct contact, fomite or mechanical vector, or intermediate hosts in which the agent multiples or develops before transmission to animal or human (i.e., metazoonoses). Examples of infectious agents requiring an incubation period prior to transmission include arboviruses, plague, and schistosomiasis (31). In the case of toxoplasmosis infection, contaminated soil and water represent a key source of infection emanating from an intermediate host (33, 34). Indoor/outdoor cats are a significant carrier/transmitter of Toxoplasma, shedding the organism in its feces (34). Oocysts from *Toxoplasma gondii* also may be transported by cockroaches and other bugs and deposited onto food and later consumed by animals and humans (35). In a recent study, eating raw oysters, clams, or mussels was identified as a new risk factor for *T. gondii* infection (36). The *T. gondii* were believed to have originated from cat feces, which survived or bypassed sewage treatment and traveled to coastal waters through river systems.

Fetal Infection Routes

Many viruses and microbes are capable of crossing the placenta. For example, the TT circovirus and several polyomaviruses (BK, JC, and SV-40) are able to cross the placenta and infect the fetus, but do not cause critical fetal abnormalities (37). In the laboratory, influenza A virus has been detected in mouse pups born of mothers exposed to influenza A virus (38). Similarly, influenza RNA has been shown to persist for at least 3 months following birth of offspring to mice infected with influenza A/WSN/33 virus during pregnancy (39, 40). A fetus may become infected with varicella (chickenpox) from its mother in the early weeks of pregnancy, manifesting as congenital defects particularly involving the cerebellum (41–43). Human transplancental transmission is well demonstrated by cases of fetal infection with rubella virus (44), West Nile virus (45), toxoplasmosis (46), and bovine leukemia virus (47).

Non-Species-Specific Infection

Mice, rats, and other rodents potentially carry non-species-specific infectious diseases (31, 48, 49). Rodents also harbor insects and arachnids such as fleas, mites, and lice that can facilitate transmission of viruses, bacteria, and parasites to and between humans (31, 49). Certain arthropods in the mite family are known to transmit blood-borne diseases like "*Rickettsia typhi*" from mice and rats to humans (49). Although mites typically are host specific, they will cross from one species to another if their choice of host is unavailable (50, 51). Fleas are capable of passing diseases by blood from rodents to humans including bubonic plague, typhus, bartonellosis, and tapeworm (31, 48). Exposure to the respiratory or urinary aerosol of rodents also poses risk for human infections (e.g.,*Hantavirus, Mycoplasma pulmonis, Streptococcus pneumoniae, Staphylococcus aureus*, and*Pasteurella multocida*) (52, 53).

The ease with which rodents transmit infection to humans likely reflects the high degree of homology between the two species.

Approximately 80% of mouse genes have a single identifiable ortholog in the human genome, while <1% do not have any detectable human homolog (54). Occupations such as farming and agricultural work that place workers and their families in direct contact with rodents and their excretions/secretions increase the risk for infection (53, 55). KIPvV and WUPyV polyomaviruses have been detected in samples from children with lower respiratory tract disease, however it remains unknown if these viruses jumped species from rodents to humans (56).

Indirect and other Intermediate Modes of Transmission

Domestic farm animals and cats that feed on infected rodents or share habitat with reservoir species may indirectly expose humans to rodent-borne pathogens (31, 53). Antibody to the rodent Hantavirus has been found in cats (53, 57–60). A case-referent study conducted in China found a positive association between cat ownership and Hantavirus infection (61). In the case of orthopox infection, cats have been confirmed as an active transmitter from rodents to man (57, 59, 62–66). A prevalence of 4% was observed in an antibody study of orthopox infection in 200 free-roaming cats, most of which appeared to occur through bites sustained during hunting of rodents (59). Compared with other times of the year, a markedly increased incidence of feline poxvirus infection has been reported to occur during autumn, when the populations of many small mammals are at their largest and most active (67–69). Human infection from farm animals and cats/dogs typically results from direct contact with infected tissues, contaminated mucous membranes, and skin wounds; inhalation of respiratory secretions; and injuries sustained from infected animals (31).

Hantaviruses have been isolated from lung tissues of bats raising the possibility that these creatures also may pose a natural reservoir for the passing of rodent viruses to farm animals (53, 70). Bats appear to play a role as well in the infection of pigs with Menangle virus (71) and horses with Equine morbillivirus (72, 73). Notably, these mammals host a significantly greater number of zoonotic viruses per species than rodents (74). Bats also have been observed to have a greater number of interspecific "host switches" of paramyxoviruses to other mammals, compared with rodents, birds, primates, carnivores, and cetartiodactyla

(74). Among humans, bats have been associated with the spread of severe acute respiratory syndrome-like corona viruses, Ebola and Marburg filoviruses, and Hendra and Nipah paramyxoviruses (74). Because of habitat encroachment and the proclivity of bats to roost in pitched roof spaces of buildings, humans are increasingly at risk for exposure to bat excreta (74).

Other intermediate modes for the transmission of infectious agents include insects and birds. Flying insects, for example, may feed on animal manure and later contaminate nearby food and water sources intended for human consumption, especially in the agricultural setting (48). Mosquitoes are known to transmit West Nile virus and Japanese B encephalitis from avian and horse hosts to humans (75–77) and conceivably may act in an analogous fashion as a carrier of oncogenic viruses between animals and humans. Lice, ticks, and other bloodsucking insects also can serve as mobile vectors to transfer neurotropic viruses (e.g., Alphavirus and Flavivirus) from reservoir host animals to other susceptible species including humans (31, 78). Wild ducks and migratory birds shed virus in their feces as they fly south in the fall, contaminating water on farms where chickens, turkeys, and pigs are raised (79).

Low or Negative Antibody Response

Viruses can induce cancer in species outside their natural hosts (80–82). However, not all viruses, especially those of avian origin, easily transmit directly to humans in nature (79). Canadian wildlife personnel, who handle wild ducks when they are shedding high levels of virus, consistently have negative viral and serologic assays (83). Volunteers inoculated with high doses of avian subtypes H4N8, H6N1, and H10N7 failed to produce a detectable antibody response, even though ~25% shed virus and had mild clinical symptoms (83). Only 2 of 27 persons in a sample of chicken farm laborers and residents regularly in contact with infected chickens and wildfowl tested positive for antibodies to Rous sarcoma virus-Bryan (RSV-B) (84). On the other hand, pigs have receptors for both avian and human viral strains and likely serve as a "mixing vessel" for genetic reassortment and subsequent introduction of genes into humans (85, 86).

Direct Human Transmission

Avian viruses can directly infect humans without passing through pigs as evidenced by the recent outbreaks of influenza A strains H5N1 (87, 88) and H9N2 (89) in Asia, and H7N7 (90) in Netherlands (78, 91). The history of human infection closely parallels the domestication of the duck, which introduced respiratory-type influenza A viruses into the "farmyard (91)." H5 subtype infection initially was detected in human sera from rural China, a region known for poultry farming (87, 92). Approximately 30% of poultry workers sampled around the time of the 1999 H9N2 flu outbreak in Hong Kong were found to be seropositive for antibodies to the virus (89). H9N2 viruses are prevalent in domestic poultry such as chickens, ducks, geese, quail, and pigeons throughout Asia (89). In Netherlands outbreak, investigators reported a high infection rate of H7N7 among people directly involved in handling infected poultry and noted evidence for person-to-person transmission (90).

Animal Infection

Influenza viruses have been found to occur throughout the mammalian kingdom in nature (92, 93) and are capable of infecting (either naturally or experimentally) animals commonly found on farms including cattle, sheep, goats, horses, mice, and cats (53, 93–95). In Vietnam, civets (a cat-like species) have tested positive for H5N1 virus (96). Inoculation with various Influenza A strains (e.g., H5N1/97, H9N2, H5N3, A/tern/So, Africa/61, and A/turkey/England/63) can cause infection of mice (93, 97–100) and cross the blood–brain barrier (97–99, 101). The naturally occurring equine H7N7 influenza virus is highly pathogenic in laboratory mice, requiring no adaptation (99, 102).

Species Jumping

The transmission route for over 200 (~14%) human pathogens remains unknown and zoonotic transfer or species jumping cannot be ruled out as a potential source of infection (1). Among known routes, infected feces and urine remain one of the most prominent modes of transmission whether by primary or secondary sources. Animals that are not susceptible to infection may still spread disease to other animals and humans if they become contaminated and share water or food sources (103). However, for domestic poultry, secondary transmission often is associated with human involvement in the agriculture setting through personnel and/or animal movement, food delivery, and the use of fomites (103). Because poultry often do not display clinical signs of infection they may not be quarantined from other animals or their human caretakers (103). Furthermore, the increasing global demand for poultry and meat products coupled with improvements in transportation, have propagated closer contact between humans and farm animals (104).

EPIDEMIOLOGY

Lack of Specific Cancer Risk across Studies

Epiemiologic evidence in support of an animal-transmitted, viral or bacterial etiology for human cancers is limited and often inconsistent with respect to specific cancer risk. For example, exposure to farm animals or manure has been associated in some studies with childhood (105, 106) but not adult brain tumors (107, 108). A prospective cohort of 20,132 poultry, slaughterhouse workers (a group with frequent exposure to avian leucosis/sarcoma, reticuloendothesliosis, and Marek's disease viruses) were observed to have a statistically significant excess of several cancers including lung [standardized mortality ratio (SMR) = 1.6, 95% CI = 1.3–1.7], cervix (SMR = 2.2, 95% CI = 1.3–3.5), penis (SMR = 8.6, 95% CI = 1.0–31.1), brain/nervous system (SMR = 1.7, 95% CI = 1.1–2.4), lymphoid leukemia (SMR = 2.2, 95% CI = 1.1–4.1), and monocytic leukemia (SMR = 9.2, 95% CI = 1.1–33.4) (7). Results of the Agricultural Health Study, a prospective cohort study of 49,884 male farmers, observed a statistically significant relative risk (RR) for non-Hodgkin lymphoma (RR = 1.6, 95% CI = 1.0–2.4) among farmers who raised poultry (109). However, in contrast to the above study of poultry, slaughterhouse workers, the RR among farmers who raised poultry was not significantly increased for either lung cancer or leukemia. Performing veterinary services also was associated with a statistically significant excess of Hodgkin lymphoma (RR = 12.2, 95%

CI = 1.6–96.3) in the Agricultural Health Study. However, an increased risk for lymphoma among veterinarians has not been observed in other studies (110, 111).

Viral Exposure

In a medical record-based study of 83 cases and 166 referents individually matched on date of birth, sex, and hospital of birth, children of mothers who had documented evidence of a clinically diagnosed viral infection during pregnancy had an 11-fold odds ratio (OR) [confidence interval (CI) = 1.1–503.2] for childhood neoplasm of the brain compared with unexposed mothers (112). However, none of the noted viral infections (mumps, varicella, herpes zoster, and rubella) were related to animal exposure. Similarly, a 2.4-fold OR (CI = 1.5–4.0, 25 cases) for childhood brain tumors (CBT) was observed in a nested (within Swedish birth-cohorts 1973–1989) case-referent (545 cases, 2798 referents) study of children born to mothers who reported a wide variety of neonatal viral and bacterial infections during the pregnancy of the index child (113). Significantly increased risk estimates were specifically observed for CBT subtypes "low-grade astrocytoma" (OR = 2.7, CI = 1.2–5.8) and "high-grade astrocytoma" (OR = 5.0, CI = 1.0–24.8). Neonatal urinary tract infections were associated with a 7.5-fold OR (CI = 1.3–44.9) for low-grade astrocytoma. This is in contrast to other case-referent studies examining vaginal and genitourinary infections during pregnancy, which did not observe a statistically significant increased OR for CBT (106, 112, 114).

Bacterial Exposure

Cancer also has been linked with exposure to animal bacteria. In an ecologic, medical geographic study, a statistically significant 1.8-fold increase in brain cancer risk was observed for countries with increasing prevalence (4–67%) of *T. gondii* infection (115). In contrast, a case-referent study of brain cancer conducted in Australia observed no difference between participants with glioma (n = 117) and referents (n = 415) in the prevalence of antibody test-positivity (35% test-positive in glioma versus 33% in referents; age-, sex-, and center-adjusted OR = 1.00, 95% CI: 0.64–1.56) (33). While it is difficult to compare the results of the above two studies given their different study designs, ecologic studies generally are considered to provide the weakest form of epidemiologic evidence (116). For example, the ecologic link between brain cancer and *T. gondii* infection is difficult to interpret given the lack of patient-level information on histologic subtype and pathologic grade. Similarly, ecologic findings of increased cancer risk among dairy farmers must be carefully weighed against the absence of antibodies to bovine leukemia virus in these populations (117).

Random Cancer Susceptibility

While few epidemiologic studies alone provide convincing evidence of an animal microbial basis for cancer, the data nevertheless are suggestive of a possible effect when examined as a whole. Perhaps the excess risk observed for some cancers, but not necessarily the same cancers across studies, may reflect a random cancer susceptibility to infection and inflammation rather than a specific microbe-cancer relationship. By analogy, animal viruses and bacteria may represent a chambermaid's master key, capable of opening all hotel doors, but only if left unlocked by the guests.

Explanation of Inconsistent Findings

Residual confounding or the lack of adjustment for factors such as population mixing, seasonality, climate, pesticides, medications, diet, and genetics may explain some of the conflicting and inconsistent results observed in the literature. Additionally, statistical results often are not appropriately adjusted for multiple comparisons and *post hoc* subset analyses, as was the case in a study reporting a statistically significant association between *T. gondii* infection and meningioma risk (33). Gene-environment interaction and the interplay between genes also are important puzzle pieces frequently missing from epidemiology studies of complex diseases such as cancer.

In the case of a "Hit and Run" virus, where the exposure theoretically occurred as an isolated event many years in the past, recall bias may have hindered the ability to establish causality or a temporal connection between a viral or bacterial exposure and cancer. A lack of study power, imprecision of point estimates, misclassification error, reverse causality, or selection bias represent other factors that may explain the inconsistencies observed across some studies and should be carefully considered with evaluating results (109, 112). Furthermore, the use of potentially carcinogenic disinfectant agents or cleaning compounds and must be taken into account as related etiologic exposures that might partially or fully explain a positive association between animal related microbial exposures and cancer.

CONCLUSIONS

While the general population is commonly exposed to animal viruses and bacteria, many of which are known to cause cancer in animals, the etiologic role of these exposures in human cancer remains speculative. For example, animal oncoviruses generally are species specific and do not infect or replicate easily in humans. Nevertheless, animal viruses conceivably may cause cancer in humans analogous to human and simian polyomaviruses causing tumors in non-permissive rodents. Epidemiologic studies to date have provided little evidence that animal viruses and bacteria cause human cancer. Future studies will need to address the complex nature of cancer taking into account multiple interacting risk factors, and perhaps a non-stationary stochastic risk that contradicts conventional research design. The latter may be especially true given the waxing and waning behavior of viruses and bacteria. The same infectious agent may present and react differently depending on a host of factors including geography, seasonal variation and climate, population density, and herd immunity. Travel, hygiene, and cultural variation in food consumption and preparation among individuals further complicate the epidemiologic study in this field.

AUTHOR CONTRIBUTIONS

Jimmy T. Efird: conception of manuscript, drafting of manuscript, critical revision of manuscript, and final approval of manuscript. Stephen W. Davies: critical revision of manuscript and final approval of manuscript. Wesley T. O'Neal: critical revision of manuscript and final approval of manuscript. Ethan J. Anderson, critical revision of manuscript and final approval of manuscript.

ACKNOWLEDGMENTS

Katherine T. Jones offered valuable comments during the writing of this manuscript and her contributions are greatly appreciated. This work was supported in part by NIH grant 2 G12 RR003061-2.

REFERENCES

1. Taylor LH, Latham SM, Woolhouse ME. Risk factors for human disease emergence. *Philos Trans R Soc Lond B Biol Sci* (2001) 356(1411):983–9. doi:10.1098/rstb.2001.0888.
2. Parsonnet J. Introduction. In: Parsonnet J, editor. *Microbes and Malignancy-Infection as a Cause of Human Cancers*. New York: Oxford University Press (1999). p. 3–15.
3. Feng M, Zhao J, Petek H. Atomlike, hollow-core-bound molecular orbitals of C60. *Science* (2008) 320(5874):359–62. doi:10.1126/science.1155866
4. Parkin DM. The global health burden of infection-associated cancers in the year 2002. *Int J Cancer* (2006)118(12):3030–44. doi:10.1002/ijc.21731
5. Tustin R. Ovine jaagsiekte. *J S Afr Vet Med Assoc* (1969) 40:3–23.
6. Weiss R. Viruses and cancer. In: Nesse R, editor. *Evolution and Medicine: How New Applications Advance Research and Practice, The Biomedical and Life Sciences Collection*. London: Henry Stewart Talks Ltd (2007).
7. Johnson ES, Ndetan H, Lo KM. Cancer mortality in poultry slaughtering/processing plant workers belonging to a union pension fund. *Environ Res* (2010) 110(6):588–94. doi:10.1016/j.envres.2010.05.010
8. Hundesa A, Maluquer de Motes C, Bofill-Mas S, Albinana-Gimenez N, Girones R. Identification of human and animal adenoviruses and polyomaviruses for determination of sources of fecal contamination in the environment. *Appl Environ Microbiol* (2006) 72(12):7886–93. doi:10.1128/AEM.01090-06
9. Lancaster WD, Olson C. Animal papillomaviruses. *Microbiol Rev* (1982) 46(2):191–207.

10. Voisset C, Weiss RA, Griffiths DJ. Human RNA "rumor" viruses: the search for novel human retroviruses in chronic disease. *Microbiol Mol Biol Rev* (2008) 72(1):157–96. doi:10.1128/MMBR.00033-07
11. zur Hausen H. Proliferation-inducing viruses in non-permissive systems as possible causes of human cancers. *Lancet*(2001) 357(9253):381–4. doi:10.1016/S0140-6736(00)03652-7
12. Nevels M, Täuber B, Spruss T, Wolf H, Dobner T. "Hit-and-run" transformation by adenovirus oncogenes. *J Virol*(2001) 75(7):3089–94. doi:10.1128/JVI.75.7.3089-3094.2001
13. Sanders FK. Experimental carcinogenesis: induction of multiple tumors by viruses. *Cancer* (1977) 40(4 Suppl):1841–4. doi:10.1002/1097-0142(197710)40:4+<1841::AID-CNCR2820400811>3.0.CO;2-N
14. Vogt PK. Avian tumor viruses. *Adv Virus Res* (1965) 11:293–385. doi:10.1016/S0065-3527(08)60549-7
15. Caldwell GG, Baumgartener L, Carter C, Cotter S, Currier R, Essex M, et al. Seroepidemiologic testing in man for evidence of antibodies to feline leukemia virus and bovine leukemia virus. *Bibl Haematol* (1975) 43:238–41.
16. Sarma PS, Huebner RJ, Basker JF, Vernon L, Gilden RV. Feline leukemia and sarcoma viruses: susceptibility of human cells to infection. *Science* (1970) 168(3935):1098–100. doi:10.1126/science.168.3935.1098
17. Jackson C. The incidence and pathology of tumours of domesticated animals in South Africa – chapter IX: short notes on glioma: and on tumours of melanin – pigmented cells, of muscle, of the adrenal, and of the precursors of the blood cells. *Onderstepoort J Vet Sci Anim Ind* (1936) 6:323–44.
18. Jungherr E, Wolf A. Gliomas in animals: a report of two astrocytomas in the common fowl. *Am J Cancer.* (1939)37:493–509.
19. Belmonte V. Über ein gliom beim haushuhn. *Virch Arch* (1935) 294:329–33.
20. Jackson C. Relationship of glioma to encephalitis in the domestic fowl, and an associated parasitic agent. *Nature*(1948) 161(4090):441. doi:10.1038/161441a0

21. Erichsen S, Harboe A. Toxoplasmosis in chickens. II. So-called gliomas observed in chickens infected with toxoplasms. *Acta Pathol Microbiol Scand* (1953) 33(4):381–6. doi:10.1111/j.1699-0463.1953.tb01533.x
22. Schuman LM, Choi NW, Gullen WH. Relationship of central nervous system neoplasms to *Toxoplasma gondii*infection. *Am J Public Health Nations Health* (1967) 57(5):848–56. doi:10.2105/AJPH.57.5.848
23. Krynauw RA, Jackson C. Presence of a parasitic agent in various intracranial tumours of man. *Nature* (1948)162(4108):147. doi:10.1038/162147a0
24. Erichsen S, Harboe A. Toxoplasmosis in chickens. I. An epidemic outbreak of toxoplasmosis in a chicken flock in South-Eastern Norway. *Acta Pathol Microbiol Scand* (1953) 33(1):56–71. doi:10.1111/j.1699-0463.1953.tb04799.x
25. Ratcliffe HL, Worth CB. Toxoplasmosis of captive wild birds and mammals. *Am J Pathol* (1951) 27(4):655–67.
26. Bartko J. [Toxoplasmosis of sheep in the lowland region of Western Slovakia]. *Vet Med (Praha)* (1979) 24(5):285–94.
27. Anderson LM, Diwan BA, Fear NT, Roman E. Critical windows of exposure for children's health: cancer in human epidemiological studies and neoplasms in experimental animal models. *Environ Health Perspect* (2000) 108(Suppl 3):573–94. doi:10.1289/ehp.00108s3573
28. Rice JM, Ward JM. Age dependence of susceptibility to carcinogenesis in the nervous system. *Ann N Y Acad Sci* (1982)381:274–89. doi:10.1111/j.1749-6632.1982.tb50392.x
29. Relman D. Chronic host-parasite interactions. In: Parsonnet J, editor. *Microbes and Malignancy: Infection as a Cause of Human Cancers*. New York: Oxford Press (1999). p. 19–34.
30. Rice JM, Rehm S, Donovan PJ, Perantoni AO. Comparative transplacental carcinogenesis by directly acting and metabolism-dependent alkylating agents in rodents and nonhuman primates. *IARC Sci Publ* (1989) 96:17–34.
31. Martin B. *Zoonotic Diseases: Institutional Animal Care and Use Committee*. Available from:http://research.ucsb.edu/connect/pro/disease.html

32. Clark S, Rylander R, Larsson L. Airborne bacteria, endotoxin and fungi in dust in poultry and swine confinement buildings. *Am Ind Hyg Assoc J* (1983) 44(7):537–41. doi:10.1080/15298668391405265

33. Ryan P, Hurley SF, Johnson AM, Salzberg M, Lee MW, North JB, et al. Tumours of the brain and presence of antibodies to *Toxoplasma gondii*. *Int J Epidemiol* (1993) 22(3):412–9. doi:10.1093/ije/22.3.412

34. Centers for Disease Control and Prevention. *CDC Factsheet: Toxoplasma Infection*. Division of Parasitic Diseases. Centers for Disease Control and Prevention (2004). Available from:www.cdc.gov/ncidod/dpd/parasites/toxoplasmosis/2004_pdf_toxoplasmosis.pdf

35. Hokelel M, Safdar A. *Toxoplasmosis*. Available from: http://www.emedicine.com/med/topic2294.htm

36. Jones JL, Dargelas V, Roberts J, Press C, Remington JS, Montoya JG. Risk factors for *Toxoplasma gondii* infection in the United States. *Clin Infect Dis* (2009) 49(6):878–84. doi:10.1086/605433

37. Shiramizu B, Yu Q, Hu N, Yanagihara R, Nerurkar VR. Investigation of TT virus in the etiology of pediatric acute lymphoblastic leukemia. *Pediatr Hematol Oncol* (2002) 19(8):543–51. doi:10.1080/08880010290097396

38. Siem RA, Ly H, Imagawa DT, Adams JM. Influenza virus infections in pregnant mice. *J Neuropathol Exp Neurol*(1960) 19:125–9. doi:10.1097/00005072-196001000-00013

39. Aronsson F, Lannebo C, Paucar M, Brask J, Kristensson K, Karlsson H. Persistence of viral RNA in the brain of offspring to mice infected with influenza A/WSN/33 virus during pregnancy. *J Neurovirol* (2002) 8(4):353–7. doi:10.1080/13550280290100480

40. Baldwin RT, Preston-Martin S. Epidemiology of brain tumors in childhood – a review. *Toxicol Appl Pharmacol* (2004)199(2):118–31. doi:10.1016/j.taap.2003.12.029

41. Laforet EG, Lynch CL Jr. Multiple congenital defects following maternal varicella; report of a case. *N Engl J Med*(1947) 236(15):534–7. doi:10.1056/NEJM194704102361504

42. Rinvik R. Congenital varicella encephalomyelitis in surviving newborn. *Am J Dis Child* (1969) 117(2):231–5.

43. Juel-Jensen BE, MacCallum F. *Herpes Simplex Varicella and Zoster: Clinical Manifestations and Treatment*. Philadephia: Lippincott (1972).
44. Lee JY, Bowden DS. Rubella virus replication and links to teratogenicity. *Clin Microbiol Rev* (2000) 13(4):571–87. doi:10.1128/CMR.13.4.571-587.2000
45. Centers for Disease Control and Prevention (CDC). Laboratory-acquired West Nile virus infections – United States, 2002. *MMWR Morb Mortal Wkly Rep* (2002) 51(50):1133–5. Available from:http://www.cdc.gov/mmwr/preview/mmwrhtml/mm5150a2.htm
46. Lopez A, Dietz VJ, Wilson M, Navin TR, Jones JL. Preventing congenital toxoplasmosis. *MMWR Recomm Rep*. (2000) 49(RR-2):59–68. Available from: http://www.cdc.gov/mmwr/preview/mmwrhtml/rr4902a5.htm
47. Van der Maaten MJ, Miller JM, Schmerr MJ. In utero transmission of bovine leukemia virus. *Am J Vet Res* (1981)42(6):1052–4.
48. Williams BH. Zoonoses of small mamals. *Clinician's Brief* (2013). 53–6.
49. McArthur J. Diseases of rats. *Rat and Mouse Gazette 1999*. (1999). Available from:http://hometown.aol.com/rattlvrr/diseasepage.htm
50. Ogg B. *Mites Medically Important to Humans*. Educational Resource Guide #27: University of Nebraska Cooperative Extension in Lancaster County (2001). Available from: http://lancaster.unl.edu/enviro/pest/bug.htm
51. McArthur J. What's bugging your rats and mice? *Rat and Mouse Gazette*. (1999). Available from:http://hometown.aol.com/rattlvrr/bugging1.htm
52. Simmons JH, Riley LK. Hantaviruses: an overview. *Comp Med* (2002) 52(2):97–110.
53. Williams E, Barker I. *Infectious Diseases of Wild Mammals*. Ames, IA: Iowa State University Press (2001).
54. Waterston RH, Lindblad-Toh K, Birney E, Rogers J, Abril JF, Agarwal P, et al. Initial sequencing and comparative analysis of the mouse genome. *Nature* (2002) 420(6915):520–62. doi:10.1038/nature01262

55. Ellis BA, Mills JN, Childs JE. Rodent-borne hemorrhagic fever viruses of importance to agricultural workers. *J Agromed* (1996) 2:7–44. doi:10.1300/J096v02n04_03
56. Foulongne V, Brieu N, Jeziorski E, Chatain A, Rodiere M, Segondy M. KI and WU polyomaviruses in children, France.*Emerg Infect Dis* (2008) 14(3):523–5. doi:10.3201/eid1403.071206
57. Bennett M, Lloyd G, Jones N, Brown A, Trees AJ, McCracken C, et al. Prevalence of antibody to hantavirus in some cat populations in Britain. *Vet Rec* (1990) 127(22):548–9.
58. Nowotny N, Weissenboeck H, Aberle S, Hinterdorfer F. Hantavirus infection in the domestic cat. *JAMA* (1994)272(14):1100–1. doi:10.1001/jama.1994.03520140030020
59. Nowotny N. The domestic cat: a possible transmitter of viruses from rodents to man. *Lancet* (1994) 343(8902):921. doi:10.1016/S0140-6736(94)90043-4
60. Zhao-Zhaung L, Hao H, Yue-Xian L. Characteristics of EHF virus isolated from cats in endemic area of Anhui province. *Zhonghua Min Guo Wei Sheng Wu Ji Mian Yi Xue Za Zhi* (1985) 5:81–3.
61. Xu Z, Tang Y, Kan L, Tsai T. Cats – source of protection or infection? A case-control study of hemorrhagic fever with renal syndrome. *Am J Epidemiol* (1987) 126:942–8.
62. Eis-Hubinger AM, Gerritzen A, Schneweis KE, Pfeiff B, Pullmann H, Mayr A, et al. Fatal cowpox-like virus infection transmitted by cat. *Lancet* (1990) 336(8719):880. doi:10.1016/0140-6736(90)92387-W
63. Baxby D, Bennett M. Low risk from feline cowpox. *Lancet* (1990) 336(8722):1070–1. doi:10.1016/0140-6736(90)92543-Q
64. What's new pussycat? Cowpox. *Lancet* (1986) 2(8508):668.
65. Willemse A, Egberink HF. Transmission of cowpox virus infection from domestic cat to man. *Lancet* (1985)1(8444):1515. doi:10.1016/S0140-6736(85)92299-8
66. Pether JV, Trevains PH, Harrison SR, Baxby D, Bennett M, Gibb AP. Cowpox from cat to man. *Lancet* (1986)1(8471):38–9. doi:10.1016/S0140-6736(86)91916-1
67. Bennett M, Gaskell CJ, Gaskell RM, Baxby D, Gruffydd-Jones TJ. Poxvirus infection in the domestic cat: some clinical and epidemiological observations. *Vet Rec* (1986) 118(14):387–90. doi:10.1136/vr.118.14.387

68. Chitty D, Phipps E. Seasonal changes in survival in mixed populations of two species of vole. *J Anim Ecol* (1966)35:313–31. doi:10.2307/2398

69. Gibson D, Delany MJ. The population ecology of small rodents in Pennine woodlands. *J Zool* (1984) 203:63–85. doi:10.1111/j.1469-7998.1984.tb06044.x

70. Kim GR, Lee YT, Park CH. A new natural reservoir of Hantavirus: isolation of Hantaviruses from lung tissues of bats.*Arch Virol* (1994) 134(1–2):85–95. doi:10.1007/BF01379109

71. Philbey AW, Kirkland PD, Ross AD, Davis RJ, Gleeson AB, Love RJ, et al. An apparently new virus (family Paramyxoviridae) infectious for pigs, humans, and fruit bats. *Emerg Infect Dis* (1998) 4(2):269–71. doi:10.3201/eid0402.980214

72. Young PL, Halpin K, Selleck PW, Field H, Gravel JL, Kelly MA, et al. Serologic evidence for the presence in *Pteropus*bats of a paramyxovirus related to equine morbillivirus. *Emerg Infect Dis* (1996) 2(3):239–40. doi:10.3201/eid0203.960315

73. Young P. Possible reservoir host of equine morbillivirus identified. *Commun Dis Intell* (1996) 20:262.

74. Luis AD, Hayman DT, O'Shea TJ, Cryan PM, Gilbert AT, Pulliam JR, et al. A comparison of bats and rodents as reservoirs of zoonotic viruses: are bats special? *Proc Biol Sci* (2013) 280(1756):20122753. doi:10.1098/rspb.2012.2753

75. Komar N. West Nile virus: epidemiology and ecology in North America. *Adv Virus Res* (2003) 61:185–234. doi:10.1016/S0065-3527(03)61005-5

76. Petersen LR, Marfin AA, Gubler DJ. West Nile virus. *JAMA* (2003) 290(4):524–8. doi:10.1001/jama.290.4.524

77. Campbell GL, Marfin AA, Lanciotti RS, Gubler DJ. West Nile virus. *Lancet Infect Dis* (2002) 2(9):519–29. doi:10.1016/S1473-3099(02)00368-7

78. Olsen C. *Zoonotic Disease Tutorial*. Department of Pathological Sciences, School of Veterinary Medicine, University of Wisconsin-Madison (2004). Available from: http://www.vetmed.wisc.edu/pbs/zoonoses/

79. Webster RG, Shortridge KF, Kawaoka Y. Influenza: interspecies transmission and emergence of new pandemics. *FEMS Immunol*

Med Microbiol (1997) 18(4):275–9. doi:10.1111/j.1574-695X.1997.tb01056.x

80. Hoss HE, Olson C. Infectivity of bovine C- type (leukemia) virus for sheep and goats. *Am J Vet Res* (1974) 35(5):633–7.
81. McClure HM, Keeling ME, Custer RP, Marshak RR, Abt DA, Ferrer JF. Erythroleukemia in two infant chimpanzees fed milk from cows naturally infected with the bovine C-type virus. *Cancer Res* (1974) 34(10):2745–57.
82. Van Der Maaten MJ, Miller JM. Induction of lymphoid tumors in sheep with cell-free preparations of bovine leukemia virus. *Bibl Haematol* (1975) 43:377–9.
83. Beare AS, Webster RG. Replication of avian influenza viruses in humans. *Arch Virol* (1991) 119(1–2):37–42. doi:10.1007/BF01314321
84. Morgan HR. Antibodies for Rous sarcoma virus (Bryan) in fowl, animal, and human populations of East Africa. II. Antibodies in domestic chickens, wildfowl, primates, and man in Kenya, and antibodies for Burkitt lymphoma cells in man. *J Natl Cancer Inst* (1967) 39(6):1229–34.
85. Kida H, Ito T, Yasuda J, Shimizu Y, Itakura C, Shortridge KF, et al. Potential for transmission of avian influenza viruses to pigs. *J Gen Virol* (1994) 75(Pt 9):2183–8. doi:10.1099/0022-1317-75-9-2183
86. Scholtissek C, Naylor E. Fish farming and influenza pandemics. *Nature* (1988) 331(6153):215. doi:10.1038/331215a0
87. Claas EC, Osterhaus AD, van Beek R, De Jong JC, Rimmelzwaan GF, Senne DA, et al. Human influenza A H5N1 virus related to a highly pathogenic avian influenza virus. *Lancet* (1998) 351(9101):472–7. doi:10.1016/S0140-6736(97)11212-0
88. Subbarao K, Klimov A, Katz J, Regnery H, Lim W, Hall H, et al. Characterization of an avian influenza A (H5N1) virus isolated from a child with a fatal respiratory illness. *Science* (1998) 279(5349):393–6. doi:10.1126/science.279.5349.393
89. Uyeki TM, Chong YH, Katz JM, Lim W, Ho YY, Wang SS, et al. Lack of evidence for human-to-human transmission of avian influenza A (H9N2) viruses in Hong Kong, China 1999. *Emerg Infect Dis* (2002) 8(2):154–9. doi:10.3201/eid0802.010148

90. Koopmans M, Wilbrink B, Conyn M, Natrop G, van der Nat H, Vennema H, et al. Transmission of H7N7 avian influenza A virus to human beings during a large outbreak in commercial poultry farms in the Netherlands. *Lancet*(2004) 363(9409):587–93. doi:10.1016/S0140-6736(04)15589-X
91. Du Ry van Beest Holle M, Meijer A, Koopmans M, de Jager CM. Human-to-human transmission of avian influenza A/H7N7, The Netherlands, 2003. *Euro Surveill* (2005) 10(12):264–8.
92. Shortridge KF. Pandemic influenza: a zoonosis? *Semin Respir Infect* (1992) 7(1):11–25.
93. Hinshaw VS, Webster RG, Easterday BC, Bean WJ Jr. Replication of avian influenza A viruses in mammals. *Infect Immun* (1981) 34(2):354–61.
94. Centers for Disease Control and Prevention. *Recent Avian Influenza Outbreaks in Asia*. Available from:www.cdc.gov/flu/avian/outbreaks/asia.htm
95. Schulman JL, Kilbourne ED. Experimental transmission of influenza virus infection in mice. Ii. Some factors affecting the incidence of transmitted infection. *J Exp Med* (1963) 118:267–75. doi:10.1084/jem.118.2.267
96. Roberton SI, Bell DJ, Smith GJD, Nicolls JM, Chan KH, Nguyen DT, et al. Avian influenza H5N1 in viverrids: implications for wildlife health and conservation. *Proc R Soc B* (2006) 273(1595):1729–32. doi:10.1098/rspb.2006.3549
97. Guo YJ, Krauss S, Senne DA, Mo IP, Lo KS, Xiong XP, et al. Characterization of the pathogenicity of members of the newly established H9N2 influenza virus lineages in Asia. *Virology* (2000) 267(2):279–88. doi:10.1006/viro.1999.0115
98. Shinya K, Silvano FD, Morita T, Shimada A, Nakajima M, Ito T, et al. Encephalitis in mice inoculated intranasally with an influenza virus strain originated from a water bird. *J Vet Med Sci* (1998) 60(5):627–9. doi:10.1292/jvms.60.627
99. Shinya K, Shimada A, Ito T, Otsuki K, Morita T, Tanaka H, et al. Avian influenza virus intranasally inoculated infects the central nervous system of mice through the general visceral afferent nerve. *Arch Virol* (2000) 145(1):187–95. doi:10.1007/s007050050016

100. Uys CJ, Becker WB. Experimental infection of chickens with influenza A-Tern/South Africa/1961 and Chicken/Scotland/1959 viruses. II. Pathology. *J Comp Pathol* (1967) 77(2):167–73. doi:10.1016/0021-9975(67)90007-2
101. Takahashi M, Yamada T, Nakajima S, Nakajima K, Yamamoto T, Okada H. The substantia nigra is a major target for neurovirulent influenza A virus. *J Exp Med* (1995) 181(6):2161–9. doi:10.1084/jem.181.6.2161
102. Kawaoka Y. Equine H7N7 influenza A viruses are highly pathogenic in mice without adaptation: potential use as an animal model. *J Virol* (1991) 65(7):3891–4.
103. Alexander DJ. An overview of the epidemiology of avian influenza. *Vaccine* (2007) 25(30):5637–44. doi:10.1016/j.vaccine.2006.10.051
104. Prosser D, Hungerford L, Erwin R, Ottinger M, Takekawa J, Ellis E. Mapping avian influenza transmission risk at the interface of domestic poultry and wild birds. *Front Public Health* (2013) 1:28. doi:10.3389/fpubh.2013.00028
105. Efird JT, Holly EA, Preston-Martin S, Mueller BA, Lubin F, Filippini G, et al. Farm-related exposures and childhood brain tumours in seven countries: results from the SEARCH International Brain Tumour Study. *Paediatr Perinat Epidemiol* (2003) 17(2):201–11. doi:10.1046/j.1365-3016.2003.00484.x
106. Bunin GR, Buckley JD, Boesel CP, Rorke LB, Meadows AT. Risk factors for astrocytic glioma and primitive neuroectodermal tumor of the brain in young children: a report from the Children's Cancer Group. *Cancer Epidemiol Biomarkers Prev* (1994) 3(3):197–204.
107. Menegoz F, Little J, Colonna M, Arslan A, Preston-Martin S, Schlehofer B, et al. Contacts with animals and humans as risk factors for adult brain tumours. An international case-control study. *Eur J Cancer* (2002) 38(5):696–704. doi:10.1016/S0959-8049(01)00423-3
108. Ruder AM, Carreon T, Butler MA, Calvert GM, Davis-King KE, Waters MA, et al. Exposure to farm crops, livestock, and farm tasks and risk of glioma: the Upper Midwest Health Study. *Am J Epidemiol* (2009) 169(12):1479–91. doi:10.1093/aje/kwp075

109. Beane Freeman LE, Deroos AJ, Koutros S, Blair A, Ward MH, Alavanja M, et al. Poultry and livestock exposure and cancer risk among farmers in the agricultural health study. *Cancer Causes Control* (2012) 23(5):663–70. doi:10.1007/s10552-012-9921-1

110. Fasal E, Jackson EW, Klauber MR. Mortality in California veterinarians. *J Chronic Dis* (1966) 19(3):293–306. doi:10.1016/0021-9681(66)90133-0

111. Kinlen LJ. Mortality among British veterinary surgeons. *Br Med J (Clin Res Ed)* (1983) 287(6398):1017–9. doi:10.1136/bmj.287.6398.1017

112. Fear NT, Roman E, Ansell P, Bull D. Malignant neoplasms of the brain during childhood: the role of prenatal and neonatal factors (United Kingdom). *Cancer Causes Control* (2001) 12(5):443–9. doi:10.1023/A:1011201524589

113. Linet MS, Gridley G, Cnattingius S, Nicholson HS, Martinsson U, Glimelius B, et al. Maternal and perinatal risk factors for childhood brain tumors (Sweden). *Cancer Causes Control* (1996) 7(4):437–48. doi:10.1007/BF00052670

114. McKinney PA, Juszczak E, Findlay E, Smith K, Thomson CS. Pre- and perinatal risk factors for childhood leukaemia and other malignancies: a Scottish case control study. *Br J Cancer* (1999) 80(11):1844–51. doi:10.1038/sj.bjc.6690609

115. Thomas F, Lafferty KD, Brodeur J, Elguero E, Gauthier-Clerc M, Misse D. Incidence of adult brain cancers is higher in countries where the protozoan parasite *Toxoplasma gondii* is common. *Biol Lett* (2012) 8(1):101–3. doi:10.1098/rsbl.2011.0588

116. Greenland S, Morgenstern H. Ecological bias, confounding, and effect modification. *Int J Epidemiol* (1989) 18(1):269–74. doi:10.1093/ije/18.1.269

117. Blair A, Malker H, Cantor KP, Burmeister L, Wiklund K. Cancer among farmers. A review. *Scand J Work Environ Health* (1985) 11(6):397–407. doi:10.5271/sjweh.2208

Chapter 3

A Qualitative Assessment of the Risk of Introducing Peste des Petits Ruminants into Northern Zambia from Tanzania

R. Chazya[1,2], J. B. Muma[2], K. K. Mwacalimba[3],.E. Karimuribo[4], E. Mkandawire[2], and M. Simuunza[2]

[1]Department of Veterinary Services, Ministry of Agriculture and Livestock, Mumbwa, Zambia

[2]Department of Disease Control, School of Veterinary Medicine, University of Zambia, Lusaka, Zambia

[3]Independent Policy Researcher, 4639 D Santa Cruz Drive, Indianapolis, IN 46268, USA

[4]Department of Veterinary Medicine and Public Health, Sokoine University of Agriculture, Morogoro, Tanzania

ABSTRACT

A qualitative risk assessment was performed to evaluate the risk of introducing Peste des petits ruminants virus into northern Zambia from Tanzania via live goat trade. Data was collected during a mission to Tanzania and northern Zambia and also from literature and interviews with experts. The risk of PPRV introduction was evaluated as a function of the probability of hazard (PPRV) release, exposure of susceptible hosts, and the consequences of spread using the following parameters: prevalence of infection, volume of trade, C-ELISA and quarantine screening missing an infected animal, PPRV viability (remaining infective) in transit, and the virus potential for infection. The magnitude of the consequences was derived from the probability of transmission and spread and the impact of PPRV introduction and establishment. Accordingly, the probability of occurrence of PPRV in northern Zambia from Tanzania was rated as "high" and the economic consequences were also rated as "high." Finally, the overall risk of introducing PPRV into northern Zambia from Tanzania at the time of the assessment was rated "high." It was concluded that import of goats and sheep be prohibited until efficient and adequate measures to reduce the risk have been put in place.

INTRODUCTION

Peste des petits ruminants (PPR) is a viral disease of small ruminants that threatens the national food security of affected countries. The disease has high morbidity and mortality rates and greatly impacts the economies of affected countries, often as a consequence of trade loss due to sanitary embargoes [1]. In the Southern African Development Community (SADC) region, the disease was officially reported in northern Tanzania in 2008 [2] and later spread to the south in 2010 [3]. The Democratic Republic of Congo (DRC) reported outbreaks of PPR that caused death of almost 120,000 small ruminants, valued at US$5.3 million from 2010 to June 2012 [4]. This did not take into account the socioeconomic and other benefits of goats and sheep to smallholder farmers [5]. In October, 2012, Angola reported an outbreak of PPR in Cabinda Province due to illegal movement of a herd of 55 sheep and goats brought from DRC [6]. Therefore, PPR is a disease of increasing importance in Africa, particularly in areas where small ruminants form an important component of agricultural food production. Livestock production is an important agricultural activity in most of the countries in Southern Africa [7] and goats play an important socioeconomic role in rural areas, especially for women who are among the most vulnerable farmers in Africa. This is because goats and sheep are prolific and require low capital inputs for a moderate level of production, reaching maturity early and are profitable to keep [8]. Until recently, PPR was considered absent in the SADC region, and as such most countries have not developed strategies on how to stem the spread of the disease in the event of an incursion [9]. It is therefore assumed that, if the disease were allowed to spread from the DRC and Tanzania into the whole of the 15-nation SADC region, it could potentially devastate the livelihoods and food security of millions of vulnerable smallholder farmers and agropastoralists [9]. In Zambia, PPR is a notifiable disease which has not been reported despite its sharing borders with the affected countries [5].

PPR is caused by the PPR virus (PPRV) which belongs to the genus morbillivirus under the family Paramyxoviridae [1]. PPRV is an RNA virus, which is closely related to the measles, rinderpest, and distemper viruses [10]. There is only one serotype of PPRV, but there are at least 4 lineages which are distinguishable by nucleic acid sequencing. The virus is not very resistant and is rapidly inactivated at environmental temperatures by solar radiation and desiccation [10]. Transmission of PPR between infected and susceptible hosts is achieved by direct contact, close contact, or through respiratory and oral routes [11]. PPRV targets epithelial cells and pneumocytes leading to respiratory lesions including interstitial pneumonia and bacterial bronchopneumonia [12] as well as bronchointerstitial pneumonia [13]. The lymph nodes are characterized by oedema [13]. PPR is characterized by high fever, erosive stomatitis, mucopurulent nasal and ocular discharge, pneumonia, necrosis and ulceration of mucous membranes, and inflammation of gastrointestinal tract leading to severe diarrhoea [14]. The PPRV is biologically and antigenically related to rinderpest virus and, clinically, the disease mimics rinderpest in goats [15]. Clinical disease is seen in sheep and goats and has been described in zoological garden collections of wild small ruminants including Laristan sheep (Ovis gmelini laristanica), Dorcas-type gazelles (Gazella granti), gemsbok (Oryx gazelle), and the Nubian ibex (Capra ibex nubiana).

Cattle, buffaloes, camels and pigs can become infected but there is little or no evidence of disease associated with their infection [16–18]. PPRV antigen has been detected in an outbreak of respiratory disease in camel and sick domestic buffaloes [19–21]. The tenacity of PPRV is considered to be low as the virus does not usually remain infective outside the body for longer than four days given the usual climatic conditions for Southern Africa. The virus is inactivated by UV light and most lipid-solvent based detergents and is both thermo- (>70°C) and pH-labile (inactivated at pH < 5.6 and >9.6) [18]. It is not well understood how the virus is maintained between outbreaks [18]. PPR outbreaks have been associated with seasonal variations, that is, more frequent outbreaks occur during the rainy season or the dry cold season. PPR is also associated with seasonal periods of increased local trade in goats [17].

The ruminant livestock subsector in Zambia contributes about 35% to the national agricultural output. The country has a livestock population estimated at 3.6 million cattle, 0.6 million sheep, 1.8 million goats, 33 million poultry, and 1.1 million pigs [22]. The Zambian livestock sector plays an important role in socioeconomic development, household food and nutritional security, and poverty alleviation. It accounts for about 36.4% of total agricultural production. About 23% of the per capita supply of protein comes from animal products [22]. Trade in livestock and livestock products exist between Tanzania and Zambia. Despite the imminent risk of PPR spreading from Tanzania into northern Zambia, there has been no objective risk assessment conducted to determine the risk of pathogen introduction into the country through importation of livestock commodities from Tanzania into Zambia. This paper therefore reports the results of a qualitative assessment of the risk of introducing PPR virus from Tanzania into northern Zambia based on the data collected in 2012.

MATERIALS AND METHODS

Study Areas

The study was conducted in 3 districts of northern Zambia, namely, Mbala, Mpulungu, and Nakonde, in 2012 (Figure 1). The districts were purposively selected based on their relative proximity to Tanzania and human and animal traffic between Zambia and Tanzania. The geographical position of Mbala is latitude 8°50.4144′ South and longitude 31°21.9522′ East, that of Mpulungu is latitude 8°46.0002′ South and longitude 31°7.9998′ East, while that of Nakonde is latitude 9°20.5278′ South and longitude 32°44.7′ East. The total goat and sheep population in the three districts is estimated at 36,662 and 1,148, respectively [23].

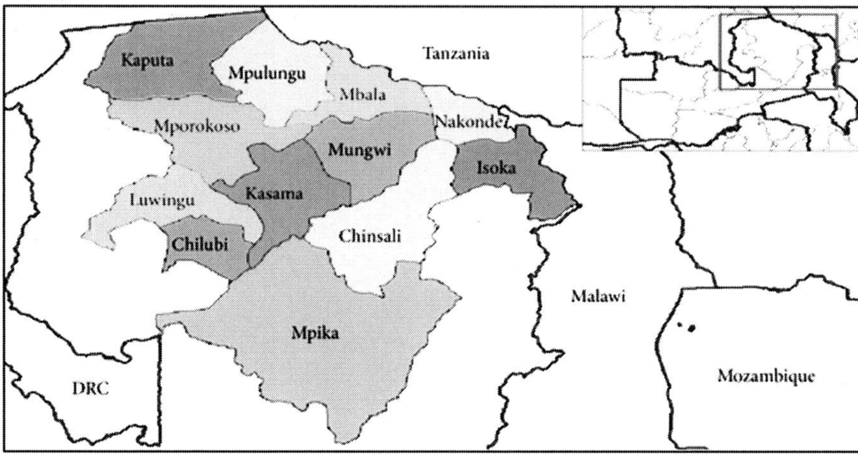

Figure 1: Location of Mpulungu, Mbala, and Nakonde in relation to other districts of Northern Zambia and Tanzania on North West. Tanzania is located in the north.

Data Collection and Tools

Data used to estimate the model input parameters was collected during a study visit to Tanzania from 17 to 24 October, 2012, where discussions were held with officials from the National Epidemiological Unit in the Ministry of Livestock and Fisheries Development (MLFD); relevant documents were obtained, and linkages to other officers involved in PPR control were made. Data was collected on disease prevalence, disease distribution, control measures, livestock movement patterns between Zambia and Tanzania, PPR vaccination coverage, and other relevant epidemiological and surveillance data.

Further data was collected through a questionnaire survey conducted along the border areas of Zambia and Tanzania from 10 to 24 October, 2012. The areas included Sumbawanga and Tunduma districts in Tanzania and Mbala, Mpulungu, and Nakonde districts of Zambia. Livestock farmers, veterinary staff, border staff, and other stakeholders were interviewed. A structured questionnaire with different sections for farmers/traders, veterinary staff, and border staff was used. Purposive sampling was employed to select initial respondents, and snowball sampling was used to identify subsequent interviewees with the help of area veterinary assistants. Questionnaires were administered on one-on-one basis with the interviewer sitting down with the respondents. One hundred and thirty-eight farmers, twelve veterinary staff working in border areas, and three border staff were interviewed using local languages (Mambwe, Namwanga, and Bemba) or English where appropriate. In-depth oral interviews were also conducted with district veterinary officers (DVOs) for Nakonde, Mbala, and Mpulungu with a focus on gathering data on livestock populations: common diseases in goats and sheep, husbandry practices by farmers, movement patterns of livestock between the two countries, surveillance methods used, knowledge on PPR, and capacity of the veterinary department to conduct surveillance.

Data from the questionnaire was coded and entered into a spreadsheet using Microsoft Excel. Data obtained from oral interviews was transcribed and transferred into Microsoft Word for further analysis. GIS coordinates were entered into a spreadsheet using Microsoft Excel. Other sources of information were from published literature, grey literature, on-line publications through internet searches (key terms: PPR risk*, PPR surveillance* PPR prevalence* PPR control*, PPR policy* Peste des petits ruminants* and specific databases such as pubmed and Google scholar) and expert opinions.

Qualitative Assessment

The methods used to conduct this risk assessment were based on the World Organisation for Animal Health (OIE) Terrestrial Animal Health Code 2001 framework and the work of Zepeda [24]. Evaluation of the following factors, both in the country of origin (Tanzania) and destination (Zambia), was also conducted: organisation of the veterinary structure; presence and capability of diagnostic facilities; epidemiological surveillance systems; disease status in Northern Province; animal population and movements; and the legal framework.

OIE Risk Assessment Framework

For import of animals and their products, the technical steps in a risk analysis as per [25] guidelines were done as follows: (a) frame the question, (b) identify the hazards, (c) model the pathway (outline the conceptual model and develop the risk scenario trees), (d) collect information (quantify inputs and impacts; probability combinations), (e) assess the risk (release assessment, exposure assessment, consequence assessment and risk assessment), and (f) describe uncertainties in the qualitative model.

The Risk Question

The question we were attempting to answer is "what is the annual risk of introducing PPR virus into northern Zambia through importation of live goats from Tanzania?"

Hazard Identification

The hazard identified is the morbillivirus causing Peste des petits ruminants (PPR) in goats and sheep.

Risk Scenario Trees

The scenario trees for release of PPR into Northern Province of Zambia, exposure assessment, and consequence assessment are shown in Figures 2, 3, and 4.

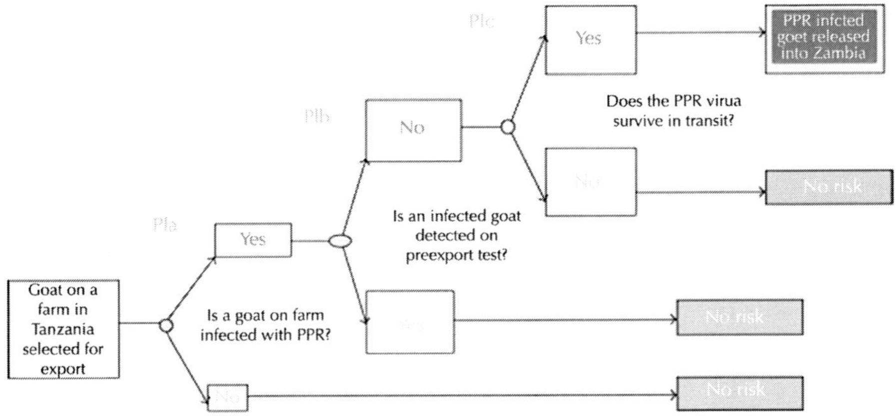

Figure 2: Scenario tree for PPR exposure to goats in Northern Zambia.

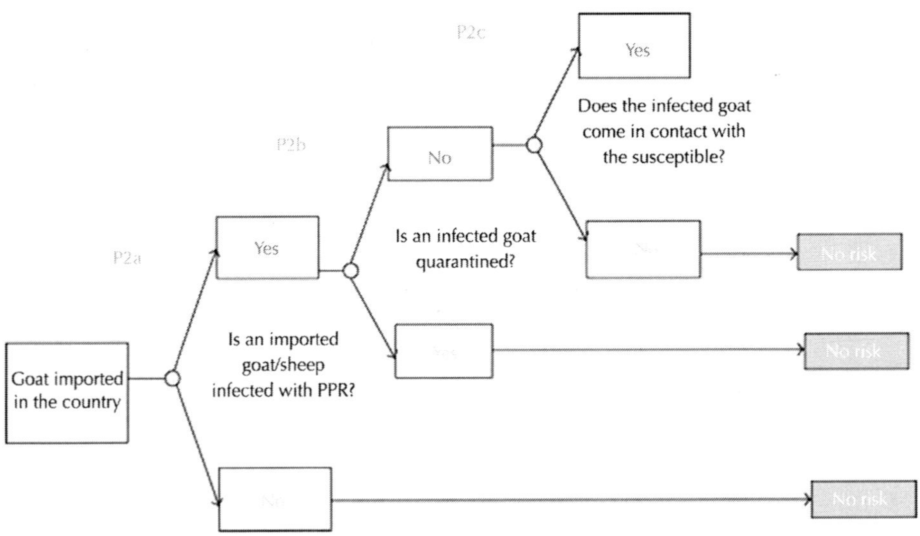

Figure 3: Scenario tree for PPR consequence of release, exposure, and infection.

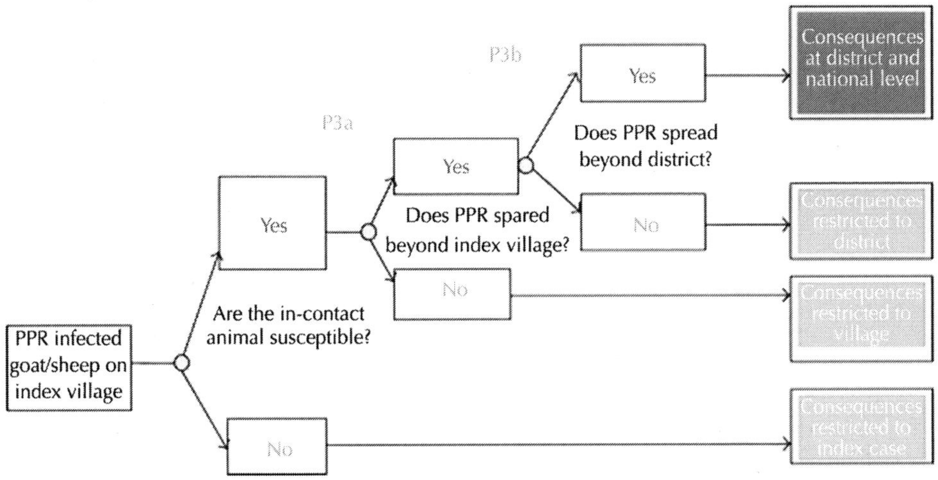

Figure 4: Scenario tree for consequence assessment.

In this study, the probability of occurrence of the risk (PPR virus infection and the consequences of the outbreaks) was equated to the probability of entry of the hazard (from Tanzania to northern Zambia) combined with the probability of exposure of susceptible animals to PPR virus. Each parameter in the assessment was evaluated based on the available information [24]. The descriptive scale developed by Zepeda [24] was used to evaluate the probability of occurrence of each event (Table 1). Combination of probabilities at each stage of the pathway, that is, release, exposure, and consequence, was done using a combination matrix (Table 2).

Table 1: Practical interpretation of qualitative probability ratings [24]

Term	Meaning for probability of event occurrence	Meaning for consequence	Meaning for risk estimated
Negligible	Probability of occurrence of the event is possible only in exceptional circumstances	Low or no impact	Allow import without restrictions
Low	Occurrence of an event is a possibility in some cases	Minor impact	Authorise with specific measures to reduce the risks

Moderate	Occurrence of the event is a possibility	Average impact	Provide assessment of mitigation options before authorising
High	Occurrence of the event is clearly a possibility	Serious impact	Prohibited until measures to reduce the risk have proven their efficiency (implement and audit)

Table 2: Matrix showing probabilities when two parameters are combined [24]

Results of the assessment of Parameter 1	Results of the assessment of Parameter 2			
	Negligible	Low	Moderate	High
Negligible	Negligible	Low	Low	Moderate
Low	Low	Low	Moderate	Moderate
Moderate	Low	Moderate	Moderate	High
High	Moderate	Moderate	High	High

RESULTS

Probability of Release

The four parameters examined in order to determine the probability of release of the PPRV into northern Zambia from Tanzania were as follows: probability of PPR virus infection of a goat selected for export; volume of trade; probability of C-ELISA and quarantine screening missing an infected goat; probability of pathogen viability (remaining infective) during transit.

Probability of Infection

The probability of infection of a goat selected for export is a function of the probability of occurrence of the hazard. It was dependent on the following factors: prevalence of PPRV from the area of origin; organisation and efficacy of the veterinary epidemiological surveillance system; diagnostic facilities; and PPR vaccination coverage.

A serosurvey carried out in northern Tanzania (Ngorongoro, Monduli, Longido, Karatu, Mbulu, Siha and Simanjiro) indicated an overall seroprevalence of PPRV infection in small ruminants of 45.8%. Highest seroprevalence (42.6–88.02%) was observed in Mbulu, Siha, Longido, and Ngorongoro districts [26]. Laboratory findings confirmed presence of PPRV in southern Tanzania by RT-PCR and serological analysis revealed that seroprevalence was 31% [27]. The official veterinary network in both countries, that is, Tanzania and Zambia is well structured and covers the whole country in terms of territory. In Zambia, districts are divided into veterinary camps run by veterinary assistants (VA's) who in turn report to district veterinary officers (DVOs). In Tanzania, the equivalent of a veterinary camp is a ward which is subdivided into villages. Wards are run by livestock field officers (LFOs) who in turn report to DVOs. DVOs run districts and are in charge of all disease control activities in their territories. However, in Tanzania, district vets are under the local government, hence at times it is difficult for the Department of Veterinary Services (DVS) to get information from them. For example, in 2009 during the PPRV outbreak, it took almost 1 year from suspicion to disease confirmation [28]. This clearly presents challenges in disease surveillance.

In Zambia, there are VAs on the ground but not all veterinary camps are manned. A number of districts face this challenge which impacts negatively on disease surveillance and control activities. Moreover, compared to agricultural camps, veterinary camps are too large for one VA to effectively manage. For example, in the study area, Mpulungu District only had one veterinary camp against 14 agricultural camps for the same territory. One VA in Mpulungu covered a radius of more than 75 Km, the furthest distance being 204 Km within the district. The staffing situation of VAs in veterinary camps was severely inadequate.

The MLFD in Tanzania had seven zonal laboratories and one central laboratory. Capacity of the laboratory staff to diagnose PPR was good as most laboratory staff were trained. Three regional laboratories and one central laboratory were able to diagnose PPR using ELISA. Recently, the central laboratory had acquired capacity to conduct molecular diagnosis of PPRV. The antibody-based C-ELISA kits, the common test that was used, were acquired from the United Kingdom though at times they faced some problems acquiring them.

Zambia has five regional laboratories, namely, Chipata, Mazabuka, Ndola, Mongu, and Isoka and one central veterinary laboratory. The regional laboratory in northern Zambia (Isoka) was nonfunctional. Out of all these laboratories, only the Central Veterinary Research Institute (CVRI) had capacity to diagnose PPR. CVRI had 4 members of staff who had been trained in PPR diagnosis using C-ELISA. The C-ELISA is used to detect presence of antibodies to PPRV in the serum by quantifying the amount of monoclonal antibody (MAb) [29]. Most commonly used ELISA kits for PPR-specific diagnosis show that, sometimes, it does not detect PPR virus antigens from some clinical samples and B95a cell derived virus. Sandwich ELISA has been developed which is able to detect PPRV antigens from clinical samples [29]. The test has undergone extensive field evaluation and has been found to be suitable for the diagnosis of acute PPR virus infection [29]. However, this test is not available in Tanzania.

Although farmers in northern Tanzania were aware of efforts being made to control the disease, only 32% had their animals vaccinated against PPR [26]. The low vaccination coverage suggests continued presence of PPR in the study area. It was concluded that there was limited capacity with respect to veterinary disease surveillance, reporting and control of transboundary, and emerging diseases which needed to be addressed in the country [26].

Based on the preceding information, that is, seroprevalence of the disease in Tanzania of 45.8% [26] and 31% [29], a low vaccination coverage in high-risk areas [28], reasonable but inadequate diagnostic capability from the state laboratories, and well-organized veterinary structure covering the whole country, the probability that any one animal selected for export would be infected with PPR virus was determined to be high.

Volume of Trade

The questionnaire survey conducted along the border areas between Zambia and Tanzania indicated the following:

(1) on average, each farmer purchased and brought (from different sources) into the flock 2 (95% CI: 1–3) goats in a year;

(2) forty-eight farmers bought at least one goat in the last 1 year (215 goats in total);

(3) goat sources: 95.6% (CI: 92.2–99.0) bought within the village, 2.2% (0–4.6) bought within district, and 1.4% (0–3.5) bought within the province;

(4) twenty-two goats were purchased from Tanzania by 17 farmers among those interviewed; on average each farmer bought 1 goat in a year;

(5) n interview of the 11 veterinary staff working on the border areas estimated that 4,612 goats (95% CI: 2,296–11,520) were imported into the country in the last 1 year.

Based on the above considerations, the probability of entry as determined by trade volume was rated low.

Probability of C-ELISA and Quarantine Screening Missing an Infected Goat

C-ELISA has a relative specificity of 98.4% and a relative sensitivity of 92.4% [30]. Sensitivity of C-ELISA for PPR serosurveillance could further be increased to 95.4% if the target population is nonvaccinated [30]. There were 19 quarantine facilities for farm animals and 28 wildlife quarantine facilities under supervision of Veterinary Services in Tanzania (Zoosanitary inspectorate Services, MLFD). Field staff in Tanzania was able to diagnose clinical cases of PPR [28]. This implied that an infected animal which manifested clinical signs of PPR during quarantine could be diagnosed and removed from the consignment and destroyed. Choi et al. [31] reported a relative specificity and sensitivity of the rapid C-ELISA of 98.5% and 93.4%, respectively. Therefore, the probability that both C-ELISA and quarantine screening will miss an infected goat on preexport screening was determined to be negligible. However, trade in livestock between the two countries was primarily informal, hence most animals were not likely to go through quarantine and screening, and hence this assessment may underestimate the risk for such type of movements.

Viability of the Pathogen (Remaining Infective) During Transit

Tears, nasal discharges, coughed secretions, and all other secretions and excretions of incubating and sick animals are all sources of the virus [32]. Due to an incubation period of 4-5 days and considering the travel period between Tanzania and Zambia (1-2 days), an infected goat will be able to carry the virus over long distances and be able to shed it to in-contact susceptible animals. Based on the evidence that suggests viability of the pathogen in live goats, and considering the short distance travelled across the border from Tanzania, the probability that the virus would remain viable during transit was high.

Assessment

Using the matrix (Table 2), the probability of release is a function of the combination of risks relating to probability of infection (high), volume of trade (low), C-ELISA and postexport quarantine screening missing a positive animal (negligible), and viability of pathogen (high); thus, the probability of release is rated "moderate" (Figure 1).

Probability of Exposure

The parameters used to determine the probability of exposure were as follows: the probability of an imported goat/sheep being quarantined (posttransit); probability of a positive animal having contact with susceptible goats or sheep on index village; proportion of susceptible contact goats and sheep; probability of transmission of PPR virus to susceptible goats.

Probability of the Posttransit Quarantine Missing a Positive Animal

An in-depth interview with the DVOs for Mbala, Mpulungu, and Nakonde revealed that there were no quarantine facilities in the 3 districts, instead on-farm quarantine was employed when need arose. The herd/flock or individual animals were placed under observation for a period of not less than 21 days. The animals were monitored by a VA for development of clinical signs/disease under the supervision of the DVO, who authorized the end of the quarantine after certifying for disease absence. The challenge with this type of quarantine was that properly fenced quarantine facilities that can adequately restrict animal movement were nonexistent. Monitoring was also infrequent. The Veterinary Department did not always provide resources at camp level to do this effectively, including surveillance. Hence the camp officers relied on farmer compliance. There was a clear possibility that mixing with local animals could still occur even when animals were under quarantine.

An interview with the officer responsible for Zoosanitary Inspectorate unit of the Ministry of Livestock and Fisheries (MLFD) in Tanzania revealed that there was little formal trade/export of live animals from Tanzania into Zambia. This meant that much trade relating to livestock between the two countries was informal or illegal. This situation made it difficult to carry out quarantine and inspection of imported goats/sheep into Zambia from Tanzania. On-farm quarantine under supervision of veterinary services for formal movements remained the only option, while informal movement's was a challenge. This quarantine was only employed in situations where the Veterinary Department had information of illegal movement of livestock. Based on the evidence that suggested lack of quarantine facilities; illegal animal movements; and on-farm quarantine that was unsecure (no fences) and poorly monitored, the probability of post-transit quarantine screening missing an infected animal was high.

Probability of Contact with Goats/Sheep in Index Village

PPRV is considered to be highly infectious, often spreading rapidly between groups of susceptible animals [18]. Infection may be associated with: the introduction of animals from another area; the general movement of animals; contact with livestock returning unsold from market; contact with traded livestock or nomadic animals (e.g., shared grazing land, water, housing); and husbandry changes [18].

The questionnaire survey with farmers and traders in northern Zambia revealed the following as sources of goats: 95.6% (95% CI: 92.2–99.0%) bought goats within the village; 2.2% (95% CI: 0–4.6%) within the district, and 1.4% (95% CI: 0 to 3.5%) within the province. As to whether the imported goats were mixed with local goats, 61.8% (95% CI: 51.3 to 72.5%) of 84 respondents indicated that the goats bought from Tanzania did not mix with the local goats while 38.1% (95%, CI: 27.5 to 48.7%) indicated knowledge of mixing. Separate interviews with 11 veterinary staff working on the border areas estimated that 4,612 goats (95% CI: 2,296 to 11,520) were imported into the country in the last 1 year. However, most of these goats were imported into Nakonde and were slaughtered in restaurants. For instance, one restaurant owner indicated slaughtering 8 goats per day. This significantly contributed to reducing the risk of contact with susceptible goats. Thus, the risk of PPRV transmission from imported goats to susceptible animals in northern Zambia was considered to be low.

Proportion of Susceptible Contact Goats/ Sheep

There have never been reported outbreaks of PPR in goats and sheep in Northern Province of Zambia. Therefore, small ruminant populations will be expected to be naïve to PPR virus infection. In Northern Province of Zambia, goats were kept under free range and chances of exposure to the virus from infected goats and sheep were likely to be high in such type of husbandry practice. Moreover, vaccination of small ruminants against the disease was not practiced; hence the animals had no immunity to the PPRV. We therefore determined that the proportion of susceptible goats in the recipient flock was high.

Probability of Transmission of PPR Virus to Susceptible Goats/Sheep

PPR is a severe and fast-spreading, highly contagious and infectious viral disease of domestic and wild small ruminants [17]. Transmission of PPR is achieved by direct contact from infected to susceptible animals by close contact or through respiratory and oral routes [11]. Up to 100% of the animals in a flock may be affected in a PPR outbreak with between 20 and 90% mortality [17]. We therefore determined the probability of transmission to be high.

Assessment

Using the matrix (Table 2), the probability of exposure is a function of the combination of risks relating to probability of the post transit quarantine missing an infected animal (high), probability of contact with goats/sheep in index village (low), proportion of susceptible contact goats (high), and probability of transmission of PPR virus to susceptible goats (high); thus, the probability of exposure was rated "High" (Figure 1).

Magnitude of the Consequences

In the border districts of Northern Province, goats are mainly kept by traditional farmers on a very small scale. Local breeds of cattle with no genetic improvement are thus kept. However, morbidity and mortality rates in susceptible naïve populations are high. Morbidity of up to 100% and mortality rates between 20 and 90% are common, except in endemic areas or when mild disease occurs [10, 33].

While the direct consequences may be marginal, indirect ones are likely to have far reaching effects. Presence of PPRV in the area may not only affect trade in small ruminants from these areas but also the cattle and the pig industries in the area are likely to suffer from trade restrictions in case of an outbreak. There is significant livestock trade in Northern Province to warrant concern over PPR incursions. Once the disease is in northern Zambia, the rest of the county could easily get infected considering the limited disease surveillance efforts in place and inadequate veterinary service delivery. Such an outbreak may be challenging to control considering there are no emergency preparedness plans in place to combat such an outbreak in the country, although at regional level, SADC could be expected to render some assistance. Therefore, the whole of Zambia could easily suffer from a ban on export of live animals or animal products. In this context, the possible impacts of PPRV outbreak were considered "High".

Probability of Occurrence

Probability of occurrence is a product of two probabilities; the probability of release/entry (P1) which was rated moderate and the probability of exposure (P2) which was rated high. Based on the combination matrix of probabilities employed in this study (Table 2), the probability of occurrence was thus high (Figure 5).

(A) Probability of release

Probability of infection "high"
Volume of trade "low"
Moderate

Test series missing infection "negligible
Pathogen viability "high"
Moderate

Moderate

(B) Probability of exposure

Probability of quarantine missing "high"
Probability of contact "low"
Moderate

Proportion of susceptible "high"
Probability of transmission "high"
High

High

(C) Probability of occurrence of hazard

Probability of release (A) "moderate"
Probability of exposure (B) "high"
High

(D) Magnitude of consequences

The probability of PPR spread within index village "high"
The probability of PPR spread beyond district "high"
High

Consequences of PPR Introduction and establishment "high"
High

(E) Risk estimation

Probability of occurrence "high"
Magnitude of the consequence "high"
High

Figure 5: The risk estimation process.

The Assessed Risk of PPRV Introduction into Northern Zambia

The assessed risk is a combination of the probability of occurrence (high) and the magnitude of the consequences of occurrence (high), and is thus rated "high".

From the interpretation of the probability scale provided by Zepeda Sein (Table 1), high implies prohibiting import until measures to reduce the risk have proven their efficiency and adequate verification procedures are available to ensure safe implementation. All uncertainties in the qualitative model were described (Table 3).

Table 3: Description of model uncertainties

Assessment component		Uncertainty description	Direction of error	Magnitude
Release	Probability of C-ELISA and quarantine missing an infected goat	There have been no formal movement of goats/sheep from Tanzania into Zambia, hence most goats will not undergo testing and quarantine	Underestimated risk	High
	Volume of trade	Most movements are illegal due to the porous border resulting in many trade routes	Underestimated risk	Moderate

Exposure	The probability of the quarantine missing a positive animal	There are no known quarantine stations in Northern Zambia. On-farm quarantine is difficult to enforce in cases where illegal animal movements are not detected	Underestimated risk	High

DISCUSSION

In this paper, we report the results of a qualitative assessment of the risk of introducing PPR virus from Tanzania into northern Zambia based on the data collected in 2012. Our design was based on evaluating the risk of PPR virus introduction through formal trade in goats. However, the study revealed that most movements of goats were informal, and we thus redesigned the investigation plan to take these into account in assessing the risk. Under informal trade, little information is captured by government officers and therefore the information provided by the veterinary and border staff was likely to underestimate the actual trade volumes and other investigated parameters. It is therefore acknowledged that there are uncertainties surrounding the probability estimates in our study, especially data from government officials.

The probability of occurrence of PPR virus in Northern Province of Zambia was determined to be high. The magnitude of the consequences of occurrence of PPRV was also determined to be high. The assessed risk was a combination of the probability of occurrence (high) and the magnitude of the consequences of occurrence (high), and was thus rated "high". From the interpretation of the probability scale provided by Zepeda et al. [24], high implies prohibit import until measures to reduce the risk have proven their efficiency and adequate verification procedures are available to ensure safe implementation. Although prohibition of import could be recommended, its implementation would be difficult since much trade in goats and sheep between Zambia and Tanzania was informal.

Therefore, risk management measures could include formalising trade in small ruminants between the two countries and strengthening veterinary services and capacity to conduct epidemiological surveillance. Since most of the cross border movements of goats and sheep were informal, there is need for the Department of Veterinary Services along the border on both sides to create awareness among the farmers of the need for government to regulate trade in livestock and also intensify surveillance, monitoring, and livestock movement controls. A joint surveillance system by both Tanzanian and Zambian Veterinary authorities could be put in place. This could help prevent the spread of transboundary diseases between the two countries, including PPRV.

Another important measure of mitigating the risk is to create a vaccination buffer/zone of 50 km from the border into the high-risk areas to avert a possible incursion of PPR [5]. PPR vaccine has been proved to be protective to small ruminants for a period of at least 3 years [17]; hence most animals will only need vaccination twice in their lifetime. Subsequent vaccinations should target naïve newly born kids/lambs. At least 85% of the small ruminant population should be vaccinated in the high-risk zone; this includes Mbala, Nakonde, Mpulungu, and possibly Isoka. If the strategy of vaccinations is taken up, there will be need to build laboratory capacity to carry out the differentiation of infection from vaccinated (DIVA) animals. In the absence of this, proper animal identification will be required, for example, ear tagging or branding of all vaccinated animals.

CONCLUSIONS

Considering that northern Zambia has a small population of goats and sheep, the actual consequences resulting from losses in terms of mortality and morbidity are likely to be minimal. However, the indirect losses far outweigh the direct losses and these should prompt the veterinary Department to implement measures to prevent any such incursions.

ACKNOWLEDGMENTS

The authors convey sincere thanks to the veterinary officials in Tanzania and the three districts visited in Zambia, namely, Mbala, Mpulungu, and Nakonde. The authors would also like to thank SACIDS for sponsoring this research work.

REFERENCES

1. P. N. Wambura, "Serological evidence of the absence of peste des petits ruminants in Tanzania,"Veterinary Record, vol. 146, no. 16, pp. 473–474, 2000.
2. E. S. Swai, A. Kapaga, F. Kivaria, D. Tinuga, G. Joshua, and P. Sanka, "Prevalence and distribution of Peste des petits ruminants virus antibodies in various districts of Tanzania," Veterinary Research Communications, vol. 33, no. 8, pp. 927–936, 2009.
3. J. Decapua, "Peste des petits ruminants in Southern Tanzania," 2010,
4. FAO, Livestock Epidemic Causing Havoc in Democratic Republic of the Congo, vol. 1, FAO, Rome, Italy, 2013.
5. SADC, SADC Control Strategy for Pest de Pestes Ruminants, Southern African Developmenet Community, Gaborone, Botswana, 2012.
6. OIE, "Peste des petits Ruminants [PPR]," Weekly Disease Information vol. 25, no. 41, OIE, WAHID (World Animal Health Information Database), Paris, France, 2012.
7. M. J. Mamabolo and E. C. Webb, Goat Production Survey-Fundamental Aspects to Model Goat Production Systems in Southern Africa-Case Study, Agricultural Commission, 2005.
8. C. Devendra and M. Burns, Goat Production in the Tropics, Common wealth agricultural bureaux, Farnham royal bucks, UK, 1970.
9. SADC, SADC Pestes des Petits Ruminants (PPR) Control and Eradication Working Group, SADC, Gaborone, Botswana, 2012.
10. S. Geerts, "Goat Plaque or Peste des Petits Ruminants," EAZWV Transmissible Disease Fact Sheet 25, Institute of Tropical Medicine, Antwerp, Belgium, 2009.

11. H. C. Chauhan, B. S. Chandel, H. N. Kher, et al., "Peste des petits ruminants virus infection in animals,"Veterinary World, vol. 2, no. 4, pp. 150–155, 2009.
12. A. W. Aruni, P. S. Lalitha, A. C. Mohan, P. Chitravelu, and S. P. Anbumani, "Histopathological study of a natural outbreak of Peste des petits ruminants in goats of Tamilnadu," Small Ruminant Research, vol. 28, no. 3, pp. 233–240, 1998.
13. N. A. Osman, A. S. Ali, M. E. Rahman, and M. A. Fadol, "Antibody seroprevalences against Peste des Petits Ruminants (PPR) virus in sheep and goats in Sudan," Tropical Animal Health and Production, vol. 41, no. 7, pp. 1449–1453, 2009.
14. S. C. Sarker and H. Islam, "Prevalence and risk factor assessment of Peste des petits ruminants in goats in Rajshahi, Bangladesh," Veterinary World, vol. 4, no. 12, pp. 546–549, 2001.
15. D. D. Kulkarni, A. U. Bhikane, M. S. Shaila, P. Varalakshmi, M. P. Apte, and B. W. Narladkar, "Peste des petits ruminants in goats in India," Veterinary Record, vol. 138, no. 8, pp. 187–188, 1996.
16. F. M. Hamdy, A. H. Dardiri, and O. Nduaka, "Etiology of the stomatitis pneumoenteritis complex in Nigerian dwarf goats," Canadian Journal of Comparative Medicine, vol. 40, no. 3, pp. 276–284, 1976.
17. P. L. Roeder and T. U. Obi, "Recognising peste de petits ruminants: a field manual," FAO Animal Health Manual 5, FAO Animal Health, Rome, Italy, 1999.
18. OIE, Peste des Petits Ruminants: Disease Factsheets, 2012.
19. W. P. Taylor, S. Al Busaidy, and T. Barrett, "The epidemiology of peste des petits ruminants in the Sultanate of Oman," Veterinary Microbiology, vol. 22, no. 4, pp. 341–352, 1990.
20. G. R. Scot, "Rinderpest and peste des petits ruminants," Virus Diseases of Food Animals, vol. 2, pp. 401–425, 1981.
21. G. Abraham, A. Sintayehu, G. Libeau et al., "Antibody seroprevalences against peste des petits ruminants (PPR) virus in camels, cattle, goats and sheep in Ethiopia," Preventive Veterinary Medicine, vol. 70, no. 1-2, pp. 51–57, 2005.
22. NALEIC, Annual Report, vol. 52, Ministry of agriculture and livestock, Lusaka, Zambia, 2012.

23. NALEIC, Peste des Petits Ruminants (PPR) Surveillance in Chama, Isoka, Lundazi, Mbala, Mpulungu and Nakonde Districts of Zambia, Department of Veterinary Services, Ministry of Agriculture and Livestock, Lusaka, Zambia, 2010.
24. C. Zepeda, "World Organisation for Animal Health Seminar on Safeguarding Animal Health in Trade in the Caribbean," Port of Spain, Trinidad and Tobago, 1998.
25. OIE, Manual of the Diagnostic Tests and Vaccines for Terrestrial Animals, vol. 1, Office International Des Epizooties, Paris, France, 5th edition, 2010.
26. E. D. Karimuribo, P. M. Loomu, L. S. B. Mellau, et al., "Retrospective study on sero-epidemiology of peste des petits ruminants before its official confirmation in northern Tanzania in 2008," Research Opinions in Animal and Veterinary Sciences, vol. 1, no. 3, pp. 184–187, 2011.
27. E. A. Muse, E. D. Karimuribo, G. C. Gitao, et al., "Epidemiological investigation into the introduction and factors for spread of Peste des Petits Ruminants, Southern Tanzania," Onderstepoort Journal of Veterinary Research, vol. 79, no. 2, pp. E1–E6, 2012.
28. Ministry of Livestock and Fisheries Development, "Trade in Livestock between Zambia and Tanzania," Tech. Rep., Ministry of Livestock and Fisheries Development, Dar es Salaam, Tanzania, Data Collection Phase of the Research Project, 2012.
29. E. A. Muse, R. B. Matondo, E. D. Karimuribo, et al., "Clinico-pathological findings of the 2011 outbreak of Peste des Petits Ruminants (PPR) in Tandahimba district, Southern Tanzania," Research Opinions in Animal and Veterinary Sciences, vol. 2, no. 4, pp. 256–262, 2012.
30. R. P. Singh, B. P. Sreenivasa, P. Dhar, and S. K. Bandyopadhyay, "A sandwich-ELISA for the diagnosis of Peste des petits ruminants (PPR) infection in small ruminants using anti-nucleocapsid protein monoclonal antibody," Archives of Virology, vol. 149, no. 11, pp. 2155–2170, 2004.
31. K.-S. Choi, J.-J. Nah, Y.-J. Ko et al., "Rapid competitive enzyme-linked immunosorbent assay for detection of antibodies to peste des petits ruminants virus," Clinical and Diagnostic Laboratory Immunology, vol. 12, no. 4, pp. 542–547, 2005.

32. OIE, Peste des Petits Ruminants, Technical Disease Card, Scientific and Technical Department, Paris, France, 2009.
33. O. M. Radostits, C. C. Gay, D. C. Blood, et al., Veterinary Medicine, W.B. Saunders, London, UK, 10th edition, 2007.

Chapter 4

Design and Descriptive Epidemiology of the Infectious Diseases of East African Livestock (Ideal) Project, A Longitudinal Calf Cohort Study in Western Kenya

Barend Mark de Clare Bronsvoort[1], Samuel Mwangi Thumbi[3], Elizabeth Jane Poole[2], Henry Kiara[2], Olga Tosas Auguet[3,6], Ian Graham Handel[1], Amy Jennings[1], Ilana Conradie[5], Mary Ndila Mbole-Kariuki[2,4], Philip G Toye[2], Olivier Hanotte[2,4], JAW Coetzer[5], and Mark EJ Woolhouse[3]

[1]The Roslin Institute and Royal (Dick) School of Veterinary Studies, University of Edinburgh, Roslin, UK

[2]ILRI, Nairobi 00100, Kenya

[3]Centre for Immunology, Infection & Evolution, University of Edinburgh, Kings Buildings, Edinburgh, UK

[4]University of Nottingham, University Park, Nottingham, NG7 2RD, UK

[5]Department of Veterinary Tropical Diseases, Faculty of Veterinary Science, University of Pretoria, Private bag X04, Onderstepoort, South Africa

[6]Centre for Clinical Infection and Diagnostics Research, Department of Infectious Diseases, King's College London and Guy's and St Thomas' NHS Foundation Trust, London, UK

ABSTRACT

Background

There is a widely recognized lack of baseline epidemiological data on the dynamics and impacts of infectious cattle diseases in east Africa. The Infectious Diseases of East African Livestock (IDEAL) project is an epidemiological study of cattle health in western Kenya with the aim of providing baseline epidemiological data, investigating the impact of different infections on key responses such as growth, mortality and morbidity, the additive and/or multiplicative effects of co-infections, and the influence of management and genetic factors.

A longitudinal cohort study of newborn calves was conducted in western Kenya between 2007-2009. Calves were randomly selected from all those reported in a 2 stage clustered sampling strategy. Calves were recruited between 3 and 7 days old. A team of veterinarians and animal health assistants carried out 5-weekly, clinical and postmortem visits. Blood and tissue samples were collected in association with all visits and screened using a range of laboratory based diagnostic methods for over 100 different pathogens or infectious exposures.

Results

The study followed the 548 calves over the first 51 weeks of life or until death and when they were reported clinically ill. The cohort experienced a high all-cause mortality rate of 16% with at least 13% of these due to infectious diseases. Only 307 (6%) of routine visits were classified as clinical episodes, with a further 216 reported by farmers. 54% of calves reached one year without a reported clinical episode. Mortality was mainly to east coast fever, haemonchosis, and heartwater. Over 50 pathogens were detected in this population with exposure to a further 6 viruses and bacteria.

Conclusion

The IDEAL study has demonstrated that it is possible to mount population based longitudinal animal studies. The results quantify for the first time in an animal population the high diversity of pathogens a population may have to deal with and the levels of co-infections with key pathogens such as*Theileria parva*. This study highlights the need to develop new systems based approaches to study pathogens in their natural settings to understand the impacts of co-infections on clinical outcomes and to develop new evidence based interventions that are relevant.

BACKGROUND

It is estimated that by 2050 the global population will have risen to 9 billion with much of this growth predicted to occur in sub-saharan Africa [1]. There is therefore an urgent need to improve food production in these regions, and livestock production constitutes an essential part of this. In addition to providing food through milk and meat, livestock also provide hides, draught power, and manure for fertiliser, building and fuel, capital reserves and cultural services and in many marginal regions is the only useful way of utilising poor quality grazing land. Livestock are key to poor peoples' livelihoods and offer an important route out of poverty.

Constraints on livestock production are varied and include nutrition, management, access to markets, natural catastrophes and importantly infectious disease (eg. [2]). Sub-Saharan Africa (SSA) harbours 12 of the 15 former World Organisation for Animal Health (O.I.E.) list A diseases considered most contagious including African swine fever, Rift Valley fever and African horse sickness. In addition, many less contagious but arguably more important diseases such as East Coast fever, trypanosomosis, brucellosis and leptospirosis are widespread. A systematic literature review on causes of morbidity and mortality among smallholder dairy farms in Eastern and South Africa identified tick-borne diseases, diarrhoea and trypanosomiasis as the most commonly documented causes of mortality [3]. This limits production directly but also ensures these regions are unable to trade animals and their products in international markets [4]. However, rinderpest is a clear example where a regional approach has produced a highly successful eradication programme and the world is now rinderpest frees [5]. This point to the need for targeted research to understand the full spectrum of disease problems in a farming system and how an integrated control package might release the genetic potential of the existing livestock while maintaining genetic resilience to environmental or emerging disease threats.

Previous work in infectious disease epidemiology has focused on single disease studies eg. Zhang [6], Bronsvoort [7] and Gachohi [8] or a few closely related diseases eg. [9] But, in reality, organisms are normally infected with a number of more or less pathogenic organisms at any one time. There is increasing scientific interest in how pathogens interact, within both individuals [10, 11] and populations [12]. Examples include studies of viruses, bacteria, protozoa and helminth infections in both humans and livestock [11-20]. These interactions can be positive or negative and involve mechanisms such as: common risk factors and transmission routes (including shared vectors); non-specific immune responses; cross-reactive acquired immune responses; increased susceptibility of immuno-suppressed or immuno-compromised hosts; non-specific effects of genetic polymorphisms and nutritional deficiencies; the demographic and behavioural impacts of infectious diseases and of intervention measures. There may also be consequences of variations in the timing and ordering of exposure, infection, and disease caused by different pathogens, including responses to vaccinations [21,22].

Animal health research in SSA has traditionally focussed on specific infections, particularly tick-borne and tsetse-borne diseases, not necessarily because they are the major diseases of cattle kept by the poor in these environments, but because they are known historically to be serious constraints to commercial systems using improved breeds. However, livestock in the tropics are routinely exposed to a wide variety of pathogens [23] whose direct and indirect impacts on animal health are unlikely to be independent of one another. Local breeds have been reared in these heavy disease challenge settings for many centuries which has resulted in selection for broad disease resistance likely at the expense of higher production [24]. Yet there have been no integrated studies of the co-distribution, co-incidence and overall impact of the major infectious diseases of livestock in the tropics. There is a need for detailed knowledge of the burden of infectious diseases impose on livestock as a prerequisite to informed decision making, resource allocation, prioritisation of research and selection of interventions. However, there is growing evidence that disease impacts cannot be fully understood by reference to single infections in isolation [25]. Instead, a holistic approach is required which considers both direct and indirect interactions between pathogens and the effects of these on the epidemiologies of infectious diseases of cattle and of the disease burdens they impose and, ultimately, of their impacts on human welfare [16, 26].

The Infectious Diseases of East African Livestock (IDEAL) project is a multi-disciplinary study which addresses two major issues: 1) the widely recognised lack of baseline epidemiological data on the dynamics and impacts of infectious diseases of cattle in the tropics; and 2) improving understanding of interactions between multiple infections and their sequelae by testing two specific hypotheses: i) that the negative impacts of different infections are not independent; ii) that 'positive' traits (e.g. resistance to infection, higher growth rates, low morbidity) cluster in certain individuals. In order to test these hypotheses we designed a longitudinal epidemiological field study to follow a random sample of newborn indigenous short horn zebu calves, with known genotype, through the first 12 months of life and to monitor them closely to identify when and what pathogens they were exposed to and the impact these had individually and in combination.

This paper describes the study design and reports the descriptive epidemiology of the IDEAL project. In particular we provide baseline data on the farm demographics and characterise the small holder African Shorthorn Zebu farming system of western Kenya which may be representative of the wider Lake Victoria basin. We also report the overall infectious disease related mortality rates and incidence of clinical episodes, the range of pathogens and exposures observed and the proportion of the cohort affected by each to provide a context for future papers on specific aspects of mortality and morbidity.

METHODS

Study Setting

There has been intensive work to define the distribution of different agricultural production systems in East Africa (eg. [27, 28]). This study focused on a specific production system, sedentary mixed crop-livestock small holdings. This system encompasses >50% of poor people (defined as income below US<DOLLAR/>15 per month [29]) resident in East Africa [30], covers extensive areas of Kenya and beyond, and is of increasing importance as populations grow.

The study site was an area of western Kenya approximately 45 x 90km covering some or all of Busia (95.9%), Teso (96.3%), Siaya (55.5%), Butere/Mumias (26.9%) and Bungoma (20.4%) districts. Each district is further divided into sub-locations which are the smallest administrative unit in Kenya for which data was available on cattle numbers. A SL typically contains 60 to 90 households per km^{2}and is 10-20km^2 in area. Land plots are typically 1-5 ha in size, with around 60% of households owning 2-3 breeding cattle grazed communally. The study site included 280 sub-locations (excluding 2 that were in Busia and Mumias towns) across 5 agro-ecological zones (AEZ). AEZ is a way to describe the type of land and its suitability for different crops and combines data on soil, topography, and climate. The areas of Kakamega, Vihiga, Lugari and Mt Elgon districts were not included as they were considered less representative of smallholder livestock farmers in East Africa (e.g. Mt Elgon slope, large-scale dairy farming more prominent) and due to logistic restrictions (i.e. the diagnostic laboratory was in Busia town, to which samples were transported daily).

Study Design and Recruitment

A stratified 2-stage random cluster sample of calves was drawn. The 1st stage cluster sample (by sub-location) was selected by random sampling sub-locations with replacement within each AEZ stratum. A total of 20 sub-locations were selected (Figure 1 and Table 1). A second stage sample size of 28 calves per sub-location was chosen at random to achieve the desired minimum sample size of 500 calves (based on logistical constraints and ability to detect a minimum relative risk of 3 with 80% power) and to allow for some losses (Table 2). A reporting system was established in each of the 20 selected sub-locations using a reporting pathway from Farmer → Sub-location-chief → Sub-chief → IDEAL Office. Each recruitment day the animal heath assistants (AHA) collated the eligible calf births for the sub-location and randomly selected 1-3 calves randomly from a hat each day. In order to be eligible the calf had to meet a set of specific selection criteria which were (1) the calf had to be between 3 and 7 days old at recruitment; (2) it was not as a result of artificial insemination; and (3) the dam was not managed under zero-grazing conditions. These criteria were set to give a reasonable window to capture calves being born without being too old and to avoid recruitment of exotic breeds rather than indigenous cattle. The sub-locations were visited on a rolling 5 week cycle to ensure there was an even distribution of calves across space and season. Calves were recruited over the 5 week cycle with 4/20 sub-locations being visited each week, taking 2 years to recruit the complete cohort. Only one calf per dam was recruited and a farmer could only have one calf at a time in the study. Recruitment was conditional on the farmer allowing access to the calf and willingness to report clinical episodes to the project and not "self-treat". A flat rate of compensation was agreed with the local veterinary office for this. Owners were asked to call the IDEAL team if a calf was observed to be ill between visits and one of the project veterinary surgeons would examine the calf and treat if considered to be seriously ill or a welfare issue. Calves were censored after any visit where a treatment was begun.

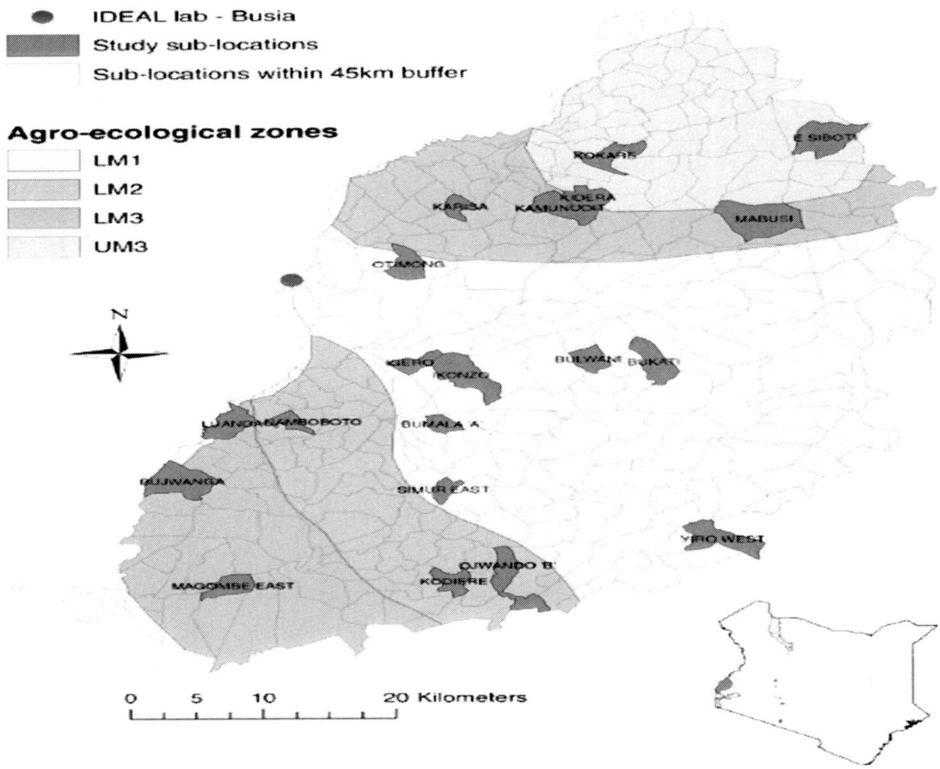

Figure 1: Map of western Kenya showing the study area, agro-ecological zones and sub-locations (selected sub-locations highlighted).

Table 1: Selected sub-locations with census/demographic characteristics (taken from the Human Population Census in Kenya 1999)

AEZ	Sub-location	No. households	Area(km2)	Cattle density per km2	Average herd size
UM3	East Siboti	1245	15.80	2439	3.4
	Kokare	325	8.29	937	6.1
	Kidera	314	7.36	728	4.8
LM1	Yiro West	1361	13.70	1187	3.9
	Simur East	415	4.32	425	3.8
	Igero	532	5.60	681	3.6
	Bumala A	724	4.38	222	2.3
	Ikonzo	1421	16.40	598	2.8

	Bulwani	478	6.87	578	3.2
	Bukati	993	11.20	1259	2.5
	Otimong	506	8.66	869	4.1
LM2 middle	Mabusi	1575	22.50	1575	3.1
	Kamunuoit	556	11.00	957	4.0
	Karisa	292	4.63	247	2.2
LM2 South South	Ojwando B	832	12.60	1095	4.6
	Kodiere	630	6.38	849	4.7
	Namboboto	351	4.46	220	2.7
LM3	Luanda	726	9.76	730	4.7
	Bujwanga	1025	16.70	792	4.2
	Magombe East	578	7.67	852	5.4

de Clare Bronsvoort *et al.*

de Clare Bronsvoort *et al. BMC Veterinary Research* 2013 **9**:171 doi:10.1186/1746-6148-9-171

Table 2: Distribution of sub-locations (SL) across agroecological zones (AEZs) in western Kenya and number selected for the IDEAL study

AEZ	No. SL/AEZ	Proportion/AEZ	No. SLs selected
LM1	114	0.40	8
LM2	86	0.30	6
LM3	28	0.10	3
LM4	4	0.01	0
UM3	53	0.19	3
Total	285		20

de Clare Bronsvoort *et al.*

de Clare Bronsvoort *et al. BMC Veterinary Research* 2013 **9**:171 doi:10.1186/1746-6148-9-171

Upon recruitment a household questionnaire was completed by interview with the owner/head of the household. The questionnaire included questions about the farm size, crops, water sources, and other livestock. The dam was examined and a form completed and if it or the calf failed any of the eligibility criteria, the calf was excluded. The calf was then examined and a recruitment form and routine visit form completed. The calf was examined for congenital deformities and excluded if any were found. This is summarized in Figure 2.

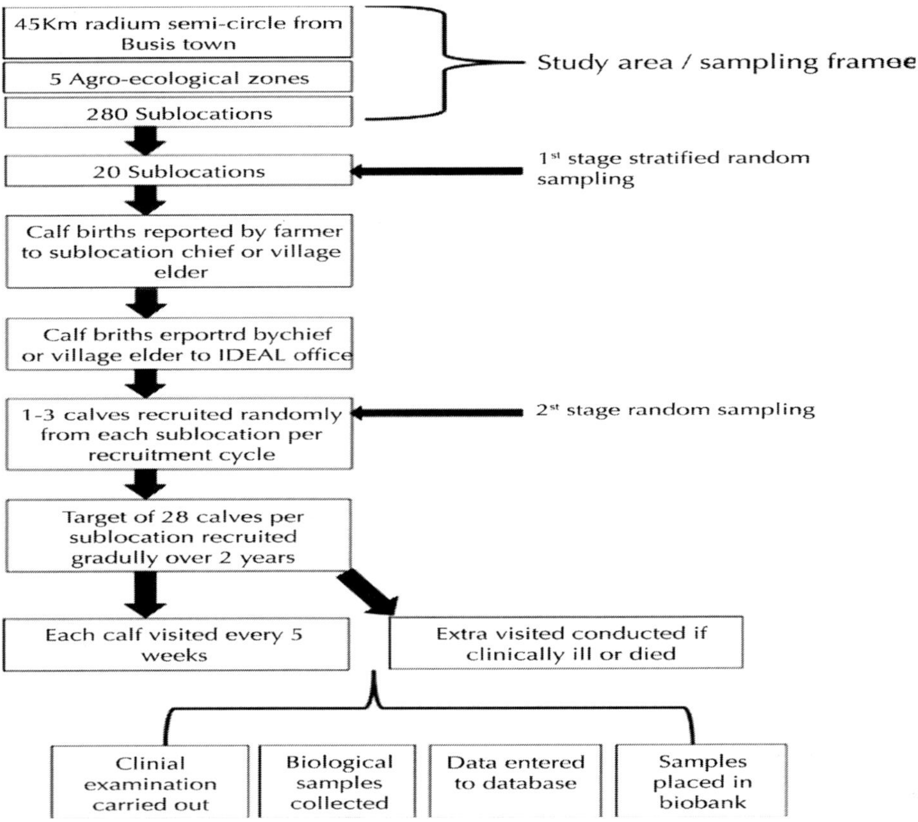

Figure 2: Schema showing the design and sampling used in the IDEAL project.

Data Collection and Training of Data Collectors

Data collection took place at the farm. A team comprising a veterinary surgeon/senior AHA and two AHAs went to each animal and followed a standard protocol for the physical examination and collection of compulsory samples. If the dam was also being visited there was an additional protocol for dam examinations. The AHAs were also trained in data collection and all questionnaires and data collection tools were piloted over about 9 months during the set-up phase of the project in western Kenya. Data were collected via a hand held Palm OS®; Personal-Digital Assistant (PDAs) and simultaneously on a paper questionnaire form. Barcodes were used to identify and link samples to individual animals. At the diagnostic field laboratory in Busia, data were downloaded from the hand held device to a database and cross-checked against the paper records and any discrepancies resolved with the AHA who collected the data.

Routine Clinical Examination of Calves

The clinical examination consisted of a systematic physical examination of the calf. This included observation of the animal at rest, posture, alertness, rectal temperature, weight, girth, FAMACHA score [31], mucus membrane colour, skin elasticity, presence and species of ticks and other ectoparasites and full palpation of the body checking for lesions and discharges. In addition to the physical examination of the calf a short questionnaire was used to update other activities on the farm such as any animal purchases or sales, treatment of the other livestock or cases of illness in other livestock.

A standard set of samples were collected at recruitment (7D), 5 weekly (5W), and 51 weeks (Y) visits as detailed below. A marginal ear vein sample was used to make a thick and a thin blood smear to screen for haemoparasites and for manual differential cell counts following shipment to Pretoria University. A jugular vein sample was collected into plain tubes for total serum protein estimation using a refractometer (model RHC-200ATC, Westover Scientific) and storage for antibody screening for a range of haemoparasites, bacteria and viruses and 0.5ml was added to RNAlater®; (Ambion®;) and stored at 4°C. An EDTA sample with 'magic buffer'was collected for genomic analysis (7D only). An EDTA sample for: (a) DNA extraction for pathogens; (b) direct microscopy on thick and thin smears for haemoparasities and (d) routine haematology including WBC, RBC, PCV, MCV, HGB, MCH, MCHC using a Sysmex pocH-100iV Diff automated blood analyser (Sysmex®; Europe GMBH) was also collected. A further EDTA sample was stored at -80°C until DNA extraction and shipping to Pretoria University for screening (Y or last visit before death) for a large range of blood borne parasites using the reverse line blot (RLB) [32]. A heparinised blood sample was collected for *Mycobacterium bovis*screening using the

"Bovigam" ELISA (Prionics®, Celtic Diagnostics Ltd., Ireland) (Y only). In addition samples were collected for white blood cell stimulation; however, this was discontinued early in the study because of logistical constraints. Faecal samples were collected via rectal palpation for screening for helminths using standard techniques [33]. Samples were divided and one part put in a plastic bag and stored overnight at 4°C for screening by McMasters technique for strongyle eggs, by the direct Baermans technique for *Dictyocaulus vivperia* larvae, by Ziehl-Neelsen stained smear for*Cryptosporidium spp.* and *M. avium paratuberculosis* and by sedimentation for fluke species eggs. The second part was stored in a pot at room temperature overnight and then prepared for larval culture to speciate strongle eggs. Samples with >2000 coccidia oocyts were also cultured to type the species of coccidia present. Three superficial skin snips were taken from the ventral abdomen and incubated directly in RPMI-1640 (Sigma-Aldrich®;) to screen for *Onchocerca spp.* microfilaria [34]. Results from diagnostic tests done in the field laboratory in Busia were entered directly in a separate laboratory database. In addition at the final visit to a calf a standard set of measurements of height at wither, nose to tail length and phenotypical measures such as coat colour and hump and dewlap were recorded. This is summarised in Figure 3.

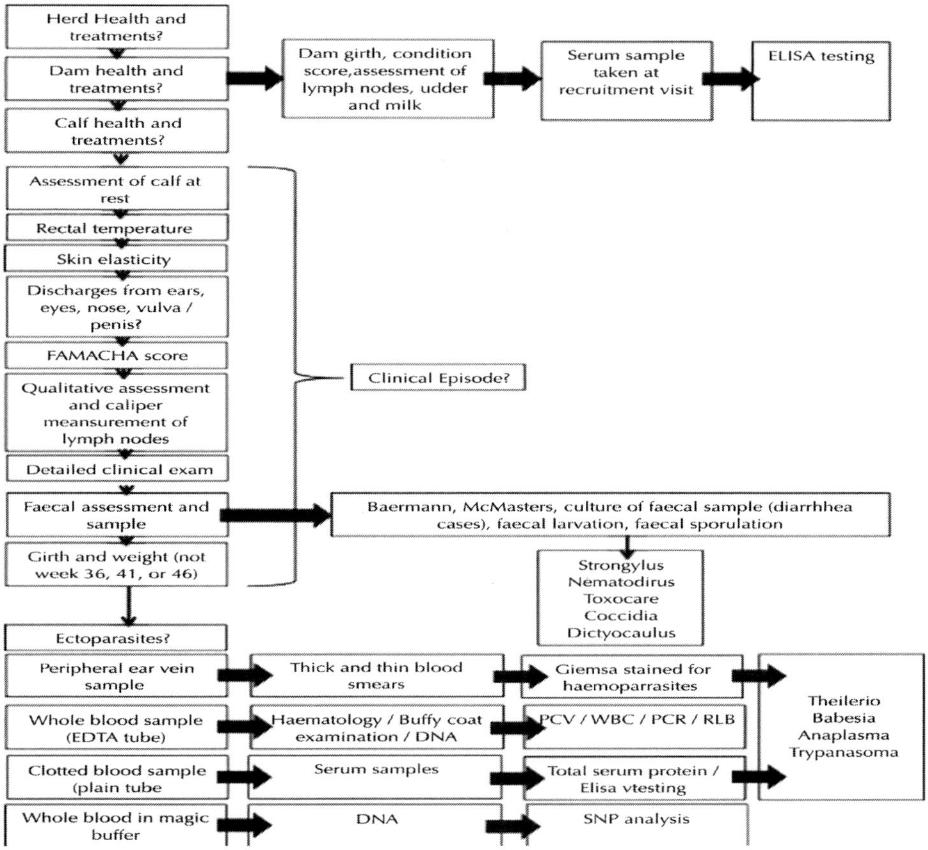

Figure 3: Schema showing the types and timings of clinical examination of calves and the types of sample collection for the IDEAL project.

Clinical Episodes and Post Mortem Examinations in Calves

In addition to routine clinical examinations and in order to capture as many clinical episodes as possible local AHAs working for the Kenyan Department of Veterinary Services in the sub-locations made weekly visits to each calf. These weekly visits involved a limited clinical examination focusing on identifying any acute disease and in particular any pyrexic or traumatic episodes. In the event that they identified pyrexia, enlarged lymph nodes or respiratory distress, they contacted an IDEAL project veterinary surgeon and an extra non-routine visit was made. The main triggers for a visit were a temperature of >40.5°C, generalized lymphadenopathy, anorexia, diarrhoea, generalised skin conditions, non-weight bearing lameness, coughing or respiratory distress. However each case report was considered and was visited depending on history and if there was believed to be a compromise in welfare. A full clinical examination was carried out and additional samples were collected based on the clinical syndrome observed. These included swabs of any discharges for bacteriological culture and typing, viral swabs and heparin blood samples for virological culture, and needle aspirates from enlarged lymph nodes for microscopy. If calves were in a severely diseased state the project veterinarian used their professional judgement and a set of criteria agreed with the ethics committee at University of Edinburgh/International Livestock Research Institute and the animal was euthanised if necessary.

In the event that an animal died or was euthanised a full gross post mortem examination was carried out following standard veterinary approaches working through the body systems. A standard set of tissues was collected from each animal, including lung, liver, duodenum, ileum and lymph nodes, with additional samples specific to the suspected aetiology where appropriate. In the event of a history of sudden death a marginal ear vein blood smear was made and stained with methylene blue and checked for the presence of anthrax bacilli prior to further examination. In the event of a positive smear no post mortem was performed and the carcass buried. If there were neurological signs and/or a history consistent with rabies the head was removed and sent for testing at the Central Veterinary Laboratories at Kabete, Kenya and the remainder of the carcass incinerated. For those animals with neurological signs and no history of possible bites, a brain smear was prepared using the standard approach for identification of *E. ruminantium* the cause of heartwater disease.

Examination of the Dams

In addition to the above the calf's dam was examined at each visit. At recruitment a full clinical examination was done (including manual palpation of the udder for evidence of mastitis), the girth measured and the animal was condition scored using a standard 10 point score [35]. In addition phenotypic measurements of coat colour and pattern, horn length and shape, ear shape, size of hump and dewlap were recorded. Two plain and 3 EDTA vacuutainers of blood were collected for possible use later. At each 5 weekly visit up to the visit after the calf was weaned the dam was re-examined, the girth was measured, the animal was condition scored and the udder examined.

In the initial phase of the study we attempted to collect milk samples from dams at each visit. These are low production animals and have very small udders and teats compared to a holstein for example. In the majority of cases we were unable to collect samples as the calf would have suckled before we arrived and/or the owner had milked the dam. Similarly the AHAs were initially trained to use the California milk test [36] but again it proved very difficult to get enough milk to test. Both these activities were suspended after the first 3 months in December 2007.

Laboratory Analysis

A full list of pathogens that the project attempted to identify that we believed likely to be present in this setting is given in Table 3 and includes 100 different pathogens. The various techniques used and the time points at which they were done are also provided for reference. In some cases there is overlap as some techniques will only differentiate to genus level while others will allow species specific identification.

Table 3: Pathogens screened for during the study

Pathogen	Test	Visits tested	Pathogen	Test	Visits tested
Actinomyces sp.	RB	CE	Hepatozoon spp. catch-all	RLB	Y
Actinomycetes	RB	CE	Hyalomma spp.	CL	7D, 5W, Y
Amblyomma variegatum	CL	7D, 5W, Y	Hypoderma bovis	CL	7D, 5W, Y
Anaplasma bovis	RLB	Y	Klebsiella ozaenae	RB	CE
Anaplasma centrale	RLB	Y	Klebsiella pneumoniae	RB	CE
Anaplasma marginale	RLB	Y	Listeria spp.	RB	CE
Anaplasma ovis	RLB	Y			
Anaplasma phagocytophilum	RLB	Y	Lumpy skin disease	PCR	CE
Arcanobacterium pyogenes	RB	CE	Micrococcus spp.	RB	CE
Babesia bicornis	RLB	Y	Moniezia spp.	FM,FC	7D, 5W, Y
Babesia bigemina	RLB	Y	M. avium paratuberculosis	ZN	Y

Babesia bovis	RLB	Y	Nematodirus spp.	FM,FC	7D, 5W, Y
Babesia caballi	RLB	Y	Non-pathogenic Staphylococci	RB	CE
Babesia canis	RLB	Y	Oesophagostomum radratium	FM,FC	7D, 5W, Y
Babesia divergens	RLB	Y	Onchocerca spp.	SNP,MIC	Y
Babesia felis	RLB	Y	Ostertagia ostertagi	FM+FC	7D, 5W, Y
Babesia gibsoni Japan	RLB	Y	Pasteurella multocida	RB	CE
Babesia microti	RLB	Y	Rickettsia spp. catch-all	RLB	Y
Babesia motasi	RLB	Y	Rickettsia spp. (DnS14) raoultii	RLB	Y
Babesia odocoilei	RLB	Y	Riphicephalus appendiculatus	CL	7D, 5W, Y
Babesia ovis	RLB	Y	Rotavirus	ELISA	CE
Babesia rossi	RLB	Y	Salmonella spp.	RB	CE
Babesia vogeli	RLB	Y	Sarcocystis spp.	HIS	PM
Bacillus anthracis	RB	PM	Staphylococcus aureus	RB	CE
Bluetongue virus	PCR	Y, CE	Staphylococcus epidermicus	RB	CE

Bacillus spp.	RB	CE	Staphylococcus epidermidis	RB	CE
Boophilus spp.	CL	7D, 5W, Y	Staphylococcus spp.	RB	CE
Borrelia afzelii	RLB	Y	Streptococcus bovis	RB	CE
Borrelia burgdorferi s. lato	RLB	Y	Streptococcus spp.	RB	CE
Borrelia burgdorferi s. stricto	RLB	Y	Theileria annae	RLB	Y
Borrelia garinii	RLB	Y	Theileria annulata	RLB	Y
Borrelia valaisiana	RLB	Y	Theileria bicornis	RLB	Y
Bunostomum trigonocephalum	FM	7D, 5W, Y	Theileria buffeli	RLB	Y
Bovine Viral Diarrrhoea Virus	ELISA - ag	Y	Theileria cervi	RLB	Y
Calicophoron spp.	FM,FC	7D, 5W, Y	Theileria equi	RLB	Y
Chabertia ovina	FM,FC	7D, 5W, Y	Theileria equi-like	RLB	Y
Clostridium spp.	RB	CE	Theileria lestoquardi	RLB	Y
Coccidia spp.	FM,FC	7D, 5W, Y	Theileria mutans	RLB	Y
Coccobacillary	RB	CE	Theileria orientalis 1	RLB	Y
Cooperia spp.	FM,FC	7D, 5W, Y	Theileria parva	RLB,PCR	Y
Corynebacterium spp.	RB	CE	Theileria spp. (buffalo)	RLB	Y

Cryptosporidium spp.	ZN,MIC	7D, 5W, Y	Theileria spp. (duiker)	RLB	Y
Dermatophilus congolensis	RB	CE	Theileria spp. (kudu)	RLB	Y
Dictyocaulus viviparous (L1)	FB	7D, 5W, Y	Theileria spp. (sable)	RLB	Y
E.coli	RB	CE	Theileria spp.	MIC, (RLB)	7D, 5W, Y, CE
Ehrlichia chaffeensis	RLB	Y	Theileria taurotragi	RLB	Y
Ehrlichia ruminantium	RLB,MIC,PCR	Y, CE	Theileria velifera	RLB	Y
Ehrlichia spp. (Omatjenne)	RLB	Y	Toxocara vitulorum	FM,FC	7D, 5W, Y
Eimeria alabamensis	FM,MIC	7D, 5W, Y	Trichophyton spp.	MIC	CE
Eimeria auburnensis	FM,MIC	7D, 5W, Y	Trichostrongylus axei	FM,FC	7D, 5W, Y
Eimeria bovis	FM,MIC	7D, 5W, Y	Trichuris spp.	FM,FC	7D, 5W, Y
Eimeria cylindrica	FM,MIC	7D, 5W, Y	Trypanosoma brucei	HCT,DG,PCR	7D, 5W, Y

Eimeria ellipsoidalis	FM,MIC	7D, 5W, Y	Trypanosoma congolense	HCT,DG,PCR	7D, 5W, Y
Eimeria subspherica	FM,MIC	7D, 5W, Y	Trypanosoma spp.	HCT,DG,PCR	7D, 5W, Y
Eimeria zuernii	FM,MIC	7D, 5W, Y	Trypanosoma theileri	HCT,DG,PCR	7D, 5W, Y
Epizootic haemorrhagic disease	PCR	Y, CE	Trypanosoma vivax	HCT,DG,PCR	7D, 5W, Y
Fasciola spp.	FS,MIC	7D, 5W, Y	Weksella zoohelcum	RB	CE
Haemonchus placei	FM,FC	7D, 5W, Y			

RB routine bacteriology, *CE* clinical episode, *CL* clinical examination, *RLB* reverse line blot, *7D* recruitment visit, *5W* routine 5 weekly visit, *Y* final visit at 51 weeks, *FM* faecal examination by McMaster's technique, *FC* faecal culture, *MIC* routine microscopy, *SNP* skin snip and culture, *ZN* Ziehl–Neelsen stain, *DG*dark ground microscopy, *HCT* haematocrit, *PCR* polymerase chain reaction.

de Clare Bronsvoort *et al.*

de Clare Bronsvoort *et al. BMC Veterinary Research* 2013 **9**:171, doi:10.1186/1746-6148-9-171

In addition, the project screened stored sera from calves at 51 weeks or from their last visit prior to death for evidence of exposure to a number of other diseases believed likely to be important in this region. Further, plasma and DNA were analysed at a number of external laboratories (Table 4).

Table 4: Serological screening tests to pathogens

Pathogen	Ab/Ag based	T e s t name	Manufacturer	V i s i t s tested
M. bovis	Ab	Bovigam ELISA	Prionics	Y
RespiratorySyncitialvirus	Ab	ELISA	Svanova	Y
Bluetonguevirus	Ab	ELISA	PI	Y
T. parva	Ab	ELISA	ILRI in house	7D, 5W, Y
T. mutans	Ab	ELISA	ILRI in house	7D, 5W, Y
A. marginale	Ab	ELISA	ILRI in house	7D, 5W, Y
B. bigemina	Ab	ELISA	ILRI in house	7D, 5W, Y
Parainfluenza3 virus	Ab	ELISA	Svanova	Y
Bovine ViralDiarrhoea virus	Ab	ELISA	Svanova	Y
Bovine ViralDiarrhoea virus	Ag	ELISA	Svanova	Y
EpizooticHaemorrhagicdisease virus	Ab	ELISA	PI in house	Y
Akabanediseasevirus	Ab	ELISA	PU in house	Y
Palyam group	Ab	ELISA	PU in house	Y
InfectiousBovineRhinotracheitisvirus	Ab	ELISA	Svanova	Y
Neospora caninum	Ab	ELISA	Svanova	Y
Brucella spp.	Ab	ELISA	IDEXX	Dam 7D
Leptospira hardjo	Ab	ELISA	Linnodee	Dam 7D

\

PI is the Pirbright Institute (formerly the Institute for Animal Health). *Ab* antibody, *Ag* antigen.

de Clare Bronsvoort *et al.*

de Clare Bronsvoort *et al. BMC Veterinary Research* 2013 **9**:171, doi:10.1186/1746-6148-9-171

Whole blood samples in EDTA were stored in "magic buffer" (Biogen Diagnostica, Spain) and were genotyped using the Illumina 50K bovine SNP chip (Illumina Inc. ® ;).

Database and Sample Tracking

The project managed data in a set of linked Access databases (Microsoft Corp.). All reports of calf births and recruitment visits were managed in the reporting database. After animals were recruited the main household questionnaire and the routine clinical visits, clinical episodes and post mortems were recorded using palm pilots running Satellite Forms (SatelliteForms.net). These were connected to the field database and daily downloaded. Every animal was tagged with a bar coded ear tag and visit sheets for each individual were kept. At every visit, the bar code was scanned to minimise recording errors. The field database generated a list of samples and then tests that were to be carried out on them in the local Busia laboratory and this was synchronised each evening so the laboratory staff knew what testing to do each day. The laboratory database linked all the barcoded samples in the field database to the respective calf, to the test results, to where the samples and any daughter samples generated from the original field sample were stored and when they were moved to the ILRI lab in Nairobi or to other laboratories outside Kenya. At the end of the field work the field and laboratory databases were merged and moved to a multiuser MySQL database that could be accessed and updated remotely giving all staff access to the data for analysis. All samples eventually were moved to ILRI Nairobi and were appended to the ILRI laboratory information management system for sample management and tracking. Samples where possible were stored in duplicate and only one of the duplicates moved at a time to reduce the risk of losing complete sample sets. At ILRI duplicates are stored in separate buildings in either -20°C or -80°freezers or in vapour phase in large liquid nitrogen biobank chambers as appropriate.

Tropical Livestock Units

Tropical Livestock Unit (TLU) is a standardising measure used to quantify different types and sizes of livestock. It gives a reference unit that captures the total number of livestock units present in a farm, with 1 TLU being the equivalent to an animal of 250 kg liveweight. One TLU is equivalent to 1 cow, 10 goats or sheep, 5 pigs, 100 chickens, and 0.7 camels [37, 38]. This unit has been used for different purposes, including calculating insurable livestock units in the index-based livestock insurance programmes in northern arid areas of Kenya. The different species and sizes of livestock kept in the farms were converted in to TLU's to serve as a proxy indicator for livestock wealth of each household. The conversion factors used here are those reported by Njuki *et al.* [39].

Analysis

The R software version 2.9.1 (http://cran.r-project.org/) was used to generate the descriptive statistics and graphics of the farm characteristics and frequencies of pathogens. All statistical tests were interpreted at the 5% level of significance.

Survival time for each calf was defined as the age at which the study calf died due to infectious causes. Animals that died for reasons other than infectious causes, or that were lost or removed from the study before one year for non-compliance were censored. These contributed "at-risk" time only up to the censoring point. All survivors to one year were censored at the time of leaving the study. Kaplan-Meier estimates of the survival function were used to determine the overall mortality rates [40].

RESULTS

Cohort Characteristics

A total of 548 calves were recruited and followed for up to 51 weeks or until they died over the 3 year period of the field work. The spatial distribution of the selected sub-locations is given in Figure 1 and the number of calves recruited as a proportion of the breeding dams in each sub-location is given in Table 2. The cattle densities in each sub-location ranged from 220/km^2 to 2439/km^2 and the sub-locations ranged in size from 4.38 km^2 to 22.5 km^2. The average herd size across all sub-locations ranged from 2.2 breeding cows in Karisa a more hilly area compared to 6.2 animals in Kokare. The life line for each calf is illustrated in Figure 4 and highlights the drop out of calves from death and euthanasia and the pattern of clinical episodes. In addition there were 2 periods where sampling and particularly recruitment were suspended. The first was following the political unrest in 2008 and work in the field was suspended for 6 weeks. This resulted in a small number of calves missing visits for one or two 5 weekly visits. The second was over an extended holiday period in 2009/2010.

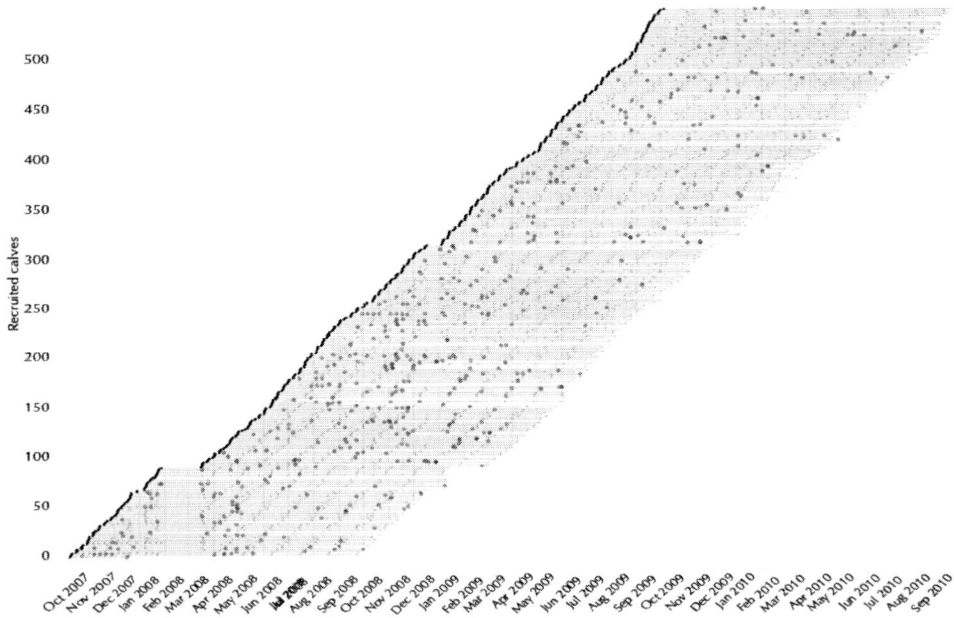

Figure 4: Life lines for each calf showing the time of recruitment, routine examinations and clinical episodes or deaths over the 3 years of the IDEAL project. Black dot=recruitment date, grey bar=weekly visit, grey circle=clinical episode; red dot= died and blue dot = euthanised.

Farm Characteristics

A total of 548 owners/household heads were interviewed. Data on the owner's age, gender, education and training level attained, and main occupation are summarised in Figure 5 and table 5. Of the 548 owners, 69% were men and 31% women. The mean age in years for male owners was 50.7 (range 22 - 85) and that for females 49.0 (range 20 - 78). Differences in ages between male and female farmers were statistically insignificant (p=0.1679, df= 352, 2-sample t-test).

Approximately 15% of the farmers had no formal education, and none had attained university education. A small percentage (21%) had gained technical skills allowing them to work in the informal markets with the common ones being masonry, tailoring and carpentry. The majority (86.2%) of the interviewed owners reported farming as their only source of income, with the rest reporting teaching, civil service, pension and business as their main sources of income with farming offering supplementary income.

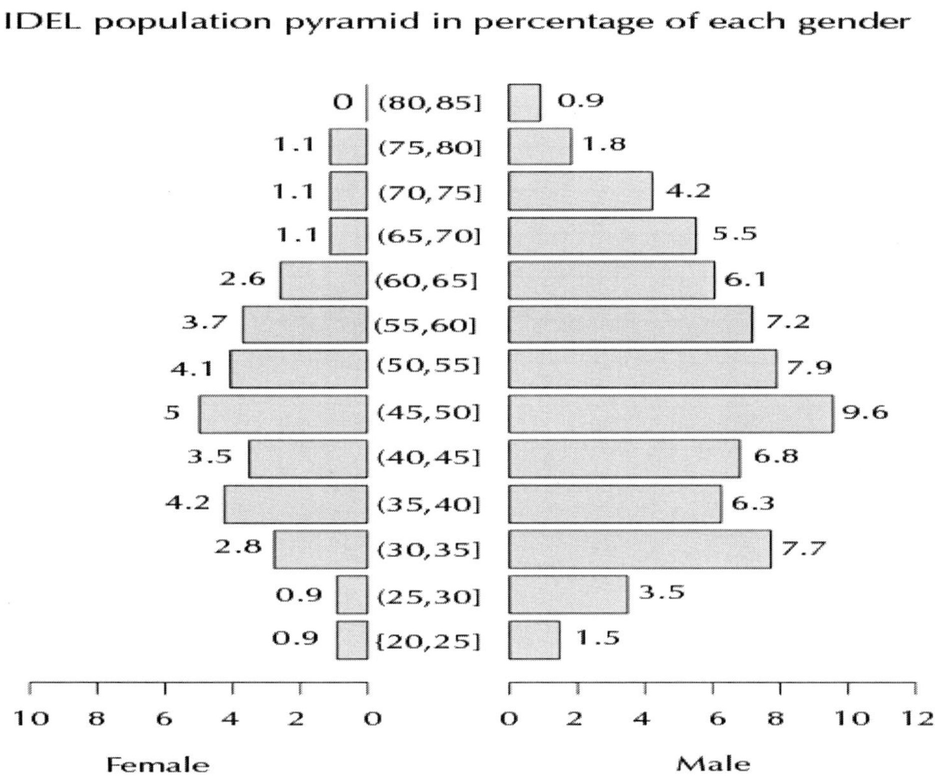

Figure 5: Population pyramid showing the age structure for male and female household heads. Each bar value represents the percent number of farmers in that age group.

Table 5: Descriptive statistics for farmer's demographic variables

	N*	Frequency	Percent**
Sex of house head	548		
Male		370	69
Female		178	31
Education level of house head	544		
None		81	14.9
Primary education		337	61.9
Secondary education		126	23.2
University education		0	0
Technical training	541		
No		415	76.7
Yes		126	23.3
Main occupation	544		
Farmer		469	86.2
Teacher		6	1.1
Civil servant		11	2
Business		22	4.1
Retired with pension		14	2.6
Other		22	4

*Not all the farmers responded to the questions in the questionnaires and N notes the number of respondents to the particular question.

**The proportions are calculated using the number of respondents to the question.

de Clare Bronsvoort *et al.*

de Clare Bronsvoort *et al. BMC Veterinary Research* 2013 **9**:171, doi:10.1186/1746-6148-9-171

The average farm size was only 1.98 ± (0.1 SE) hectares (range 0.1 to 23.1 ha), with majority (96.1%) being owned. Such land is continuously sub-divided, to give adult sons an inheritance and ownership rights. This practice results in families owning small pieces of land that are sometimes not economically viable for agriculture. The rest (3.9%) rented the land they farmed on. All the farms selected for the study kept cattle and also planted food crops, with each farm having a median 5 (range 1 to 131) cattle. The indigenous short horn zebu cattle were the predominant breed kept, with only a small percentage

(3.1%) also keeping zebu crosses. Farmers kept more than one species of livestock; an attribute identified as a strategy for spreading risk of losses [41, 42]. Different livestock species serve different purposes within the farm enterprise. The general herd structure is given in Table 6, with adult females comprising 41.4% of all cattle kept, and adult males 9.8%.

Table 6: Land sizes, livestock species kept and the herd structure

	N	Percent	Mean	median	s.d.	Min.	Max.
Land size owned (hectares)							
	517	94.3	1.98	1.37	2.28	0.1	23.1
Livestock numbers							
All cattle	548	100	6.5	5	7.6	1	131
Indigenous cattle	548	100	6.5	5	7.6	1	131
Cross breds	17	3.1	1.4	1	1	1	5
Goats	209	38.1	3.5	3	3.8	1	33
Sheep	112	20.4	3.9	2.5	5.3	1	48
Pigs	150	27.3	2.2	1	2.2	1	13
Chickens	485	88.5	14.3	10	12.7	1	120
Dogs	297	54.2	2.04	2	1.4	1	9
Tropical livestock units	546	99.6	5.8	4.1	6.71	0.48	114.3
Herd structure (indigenous)	548	Frequency	Mean/farm	Percent			
Adult females		1463	2.7	41.4			
Adult males		345	0.6	9.8			
Female calves		465	0.8	13.2			
Male calves		446	0.8	12.6			
Weaning females		399	0.7	11.3			
Weaning males		417	0.8	11.8			
Total		3535	6.5	100.0			

de Clare Bronsvoort *et al.*

de Clare Bronsvoort *et al.* *BMC Veterinary Research* 2013 **9**:171, doi:10.1186/1746-6148-9-171

Husbandry and Management Practices

Almost 60% of the farms provided housing for livestock. This was usually in the form of an open yard/kraal surrounded by a fence made of untreated wood or bushes with no roof. The remaining 40% of farms provided no housing and the animals were left free or tethered within the homestead during the night. Among those providing housing, 83.1% housed calves separate from the dams/bulls. Calves were not allowed to graze with adults (in 94.4% of the farms) until after weaning. This was mainly to prevent calves suckling dams while out in the field. Calves were allowed to suckle as the farmer milked, with some farmers reporting that milk-let-down in their short horn zebus only happened when stimulated by calves. Other farmers obtained their share first and left the rest for the calf to suckle.

During the dry season, 49.1% of the farms reported providing drinking water for the cattle within the homestead. The rest drove their animals to a water source. These proportions did not differ significantly between the dry and the wet seasons. Distances to the watering points were below 1 km for 73.8% and 75.8% of the farms in the dry and wet seasons respectively, with the rest travelling more than 1 km to access drinking water. Table 7 shows data on the housing, distances to watering points, frequency of watering, and quality of water both in the dry and wet seasons.

Table 7: Description of housing, and watering practices in the dry and wet seasons

	N	Dryseason		Wet season	
Housing	545	Freq	Percent	Freq	Percent
Kraal/yard		321	58.9	322.0	59.3
None		224	41.1	223.0	40.7
Access to water	547				
Distance to furthest					
watering point					

At homestead		91	16.6	100.0	18.3
<1 km		313	57.2	314.0	57.5
1–5 km		141	25.8	131.0	24
6–10 km		2	0.4	1.0	0.2
Frequency of					
watering					
Freely available		11	2	13.0	2.4
Once a day		149	27.2	446.0	81.5
Twice a day		367	67.1	87.0	15.9
Thrice a day		20	3.7	1.0	0.2
Water quality					
Good, clear		533	97.4	508.0	92.9
Muddy		14	2.6	39.0	7.1

de Clare Bronsvoort *et al.*

de Clare Bronsvoort *et al. BMC Veterinary Research* 2013 9:171, doi:10.1186/1746-6148-9-171

Cattle Trading and Breeding Practices

Almost all the cattle purchases and sales (98.9%) were done through cattle markets (Table 8). The rest (1.1%) of the farms reported trading animals directly with neighboring farms. A total of 24 different cattle markets were reported serving the 20 sub-locations, spanning four administrative districts. However, a quarter (6/24) of these markets served 71.2% of all the farmers in the study, an indication that farmers preferred trading in big markets, where they are likely to get more competitive prices.

Table 8: Location of trading markets and sources of breeding bulls

	N	Freq	Percent
Location of	504		
purchasing point			
Within sublocation		75	14.9

Neighbouring sublocation		396	78.6
Other		33	6.5
Purchasing point	539		
Market		533	98.9
Neighbouring farm		6	1.1
Breeding practices	548		
Own bull (bred)		63	11.5
Own bull (bought)		45	8.2
Bull donated		2	0.4
Bull borrowed		422	77
Communal area bull		19	3.5
Other		1	0.1

de Clare Bronsvoort *et al.*

de Clare Bronsvoort *et al. BMC Veterinary Research* 2013 **9**:171, doi:10.1186/1746-6148-9-171

There were no reports of organized breeding programmes, and farmers did not keep any written breeding records. The choice of breeding bulls was mostly based on availability of a bull, and if more than one then the farmer decided on personal preferences. Only 11.4% and 8.2% of the farms kept own-bred or purchased breeding bulls respectively (see table 8). Most farmers (76.2%) borrowed breeding bulls whenever their cows needed service. Based on this, only a few bulls are available to serve animals, raising the chances of widespread inbreeding. A few farmers (3.4%) indicated they did not make any direct breeding decisions and depended on their cows being served while grazing in the same communal areas or at watering points. This number is likely to be much higher than reported as animals mix freely and frequently at watering points and communal grazing fields.

Access to Veterinary Services

During the farmer interview at the recruitment visit, most farmers (84.7%) reported accessing some form of veterinary services, mainly provided by private animal health workers, and to a lesser extent by government animal health workers, and veterinary drug suppliers (see Table 9). A few farmers indicated they did not use the services of an animal health worker, and instead treated their sick animals themselves. Approximately 90% of farmers reported using some form of tick control of which most (89.9%) reported using whole body spraying with acaricides at the farm. Only a few farmers reported accessing communal cattle dips. Most of the cattle dips in the study sub-locations are abandoned and not in use. Only just over 50% of farmers reported using any form of anthelminthic treatment and only around 18% reported using any form of tsetse control. A moderate proportion of farmers reported using vaccination (52%) although most of those reporting using vaccines did not know what vaccine they had given their animals or what they were protected against (76.7%) and their use seems to be largely driven by need rather than a regular programme of control.

Table 9: Description of access to veterinary services and disease control practices in the farm as reported during the calf recruitment visit

		Frequency	Percent
Access to veterinary services	544		
Yes		461	84.7
No		83	15.3
Type of Veterinary support	461		
Private animal health worker		264	57.3
Government animal health worker		176	38.2
Veterinary drug supplier		23	5.0
Farmer		10	2.2
Tick-control	548		
Yes		498	90.9
No		50	9.1
Application method	498		
Spraying whole body		462	92.7
Spraying legs only		9	1.8
Pour on		6	1.2
Hand dressing		25	5.0
Dipping		8	1.6
Other (traditional,manual removal)		10	2

Worm control	548		
Yes		309	56.4
No		239	43.6
Application method	309		
Drench		265	85.8
Bollet		47	15.2
Others (injectables/unknown)		2	0.6
Traditional		5	1.6
Trypanosome control	548		
Yes		98	17.9
No		450	82.1
Method used	98		
Spraying whole body		51	52.0
Chemotherapy		32	32.7
Pour-on		10	10.2
Other (dipping/head dressing/			
unknown)		8	8.2
Use of Vaccines	546		
Yes		284	52.0
No		262	48.0
Frequency of use	277		
Routinely		9	2.9
When need arises		269	97.1
Vaccine type used	284		
Unknown		230	81.0
Anthrax		8	2.8
Black quarter		11	3.9
Contagious Bovine Pleural Pneumonia		1	0.4
Foot and mouth disease		25	8.8
Lumpy skin disease		18	6.3
Other		6	2.1

de Clare Bronsvoort *et al.*

de Clare Bronsvoort *et al.* *BMC Veterinary Research* 2013 **9**:171, doi:10.1186/1746-6148-9-171

There was a notable difference between the proportion of farmers who reported carrying out disease control measures such as tick control and worming during the initial visit, and the actual proportion of farmers who reported using any preventive measures during the one year follow up period. This suggests that farmers are answering what they think they should be doing or maybe have done but a significant proportion actually then appeared to not carry out these measures over the course of our observations. Interestingly with tsetse control stated and observed activities seem to align well possibly reflecting the recent inputs form NGOs in this area. In contrast vaccination use was much higher than stated and this is not clear why such a discrepancy should arise. This highlights the need for caution in interpreting responses especially from cross-sectional data (see Table 10).

Table 10: Table comparing the proportion of farms reporting using each disease control measure at initial visit alongside actual proportion of farms that carried out the measures during the follow up period (n = 548)

Type of control	Initial visit %	Actual practice %
Tick control*		
Yes	90.9	69.9
No	9.1	30.1
Worm control*		
Yes	56.4	26.8
No	43.6	73.2
Tsetse and trypanosome control		
Yes	17.9	14.1
No	82.1	85.9
Vaccine use*		
Yes	52.0	96.4
No	48.0	3.6

*significantly different at the 5% level using a McNemar's chi-squared test.

de Clare Bronsvoort *et al.*

de Clare Bronsvoort *et al.* *BMC Veterinary Research* 2013 **9**:171, doi:10.1186/1746-6148-9-171

Morbidity and Mortality

The 548 recruited calves contributed a total of 175,732 calf days of life to the study. Figure 4 shows the temporal pattern of deaths and clinical episodes over the 3 years of the study. A total of 88 calves died before reaching 51 weeks of age giving an crude mortality rate of 16.4 (13.2-19.5) per 100 calves in their first year of life (Table 11).

Table 11: Counts of primary cause of deaths attributed by expert committee

Cause of death	No. calves
East coast fever	32
Unknown	20
Haemonchosis	9
Heartwater	6
Trauma	3
Actiomyces pyogenes	1
Babesiosis	1
Bacterialpneumonia	1
Black Quarter	1
Cassava	1
Foreign body	1
Mis-mothering	1
Rabies	1
Salmonellosis	1
Trypanosomiasis	1
Turning sickness	1
Viral pneumonia	1
No post mortem carried out	6
Total	88

NB 2 additional calves were considered to have died with ECF as a secondary contributing cause; one with heartwater and another with black quarter.

de Clare Bronsvoort *et al.*

de Clare Bronsvoort *et al.* *BMC Veterinary Research* 2013 **9**:171, doi:10.1186/1746-6148-9-171

Fifteen calves were euthanised and were considered to have died from the primary pathology reported on *post mortem*. The distribution of times of deaths by AEZ is given in the Kaplan-Meier plot (Figure 6) showing that AEZ5 which is UM3 in Figure 1 and includes Magombe East, followed by AEZ1 (LM1) which includes Bumala A had much higher death rates than other AEZs. The reasons are not yet clear and are the subject of ongoing analyses. Deaths were also attributed to a secondary or contributing cause of death when this was appropriate.

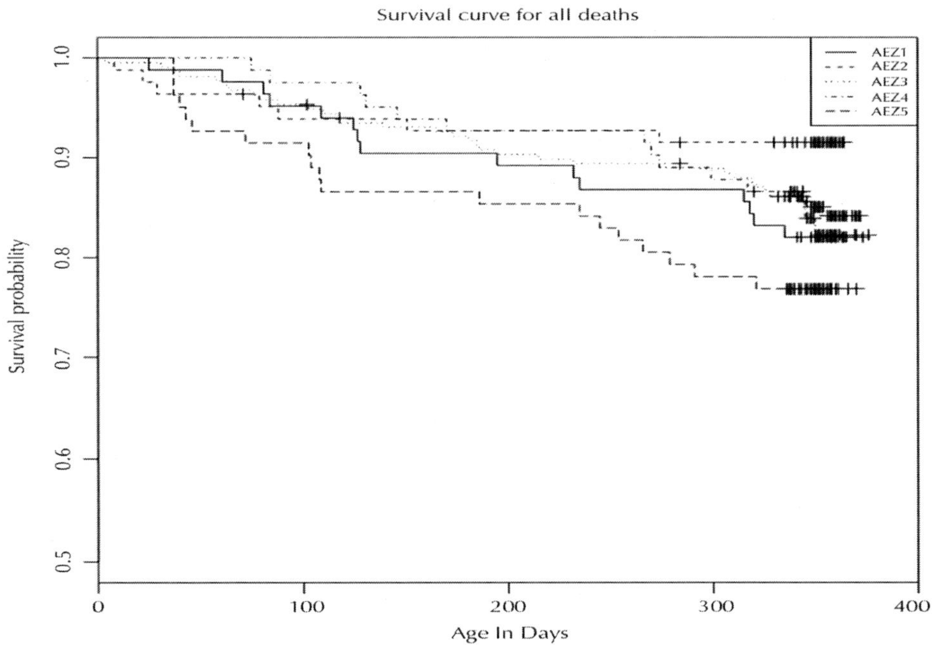

Figure 6: Kaplan-Meier survival curves for deaths due to all causes.+ mark censoring for reasons other than death and are mainly at 51 weeks when visits stopped. The dashed lines give the 95% confidence intervals on the survival probability.

Unfortunately due to logistical reasons *post mortems* were not carried out on 6 of these calves so their cause of death remained unknown. Of the remaining 82 deaths all received a post-mortem examination. A further 4 of this 82 were of unknown cause (a total of 10 calves that died of a completely unknown cause). Seven died from a known non-infectious cause (cassava poisoning (1), foreign body pneumonia (1), mismothering (1), starvation (1), trauma (3)) and 1 died from an unidentified non-infectious cause. Eleven calves had clinical signs indicative of an infectious agent but the definitive cause remained unidentified and 59 died of an infectious cause that was diagnosed by post-mortem examination, appropriate testing and clinical history (East Coast fever (33), turning sickness (1), haemonchosis (10), heartwater (6), babesiosis (1), rabies (1), salmonellosis (1), trypanosomiasis (1), black quarter (1), viral pneumonia (1), multifocal abcessation due to*Actinomyces pyogenes* (1), and *Arcanobacterium* infection (1). This gives a minimum of 70 deaths attributable to infectious diseases and a minimum mortality rate due to infectious causes of 13.3% (10.4-16.2) per 100 calves in the first year of life.

Of the 32 cases of East Coast Fever 8 had a contributing cause of helminthiasis, 5 of which were due to haemonchosis and 2 of trypanosomiasis. Of the 10 cases of haemonchosis 2 had a contributing cause of Theileriosis, and 1 of lung worm (*Dictyocaulus viviparous*). Of the 6 heartwater cases 1 had a contributing cause of East Coast fever as did the case of black quarter. It is interesting to note that in an area generally considered to have high tsetse challenge there seemed to be little clinical trypanosomiasis.

A further 307 clinical episodes were observed by the AHAs on their routine 5 weekly visits and 216 clinical episodes were reported during non-routine visits in response to reported illness. The details of all the clinical signs and patterns is currently under analysis but the overall distribution of clinical episodes by age is given in Figure 7. This suggests a bimodal pattern with a large peak around 16 weeks at the time when maternal antibodies might be expected to be waning. There is a second smaller peak later around 41 weeks when many calves are weaned.

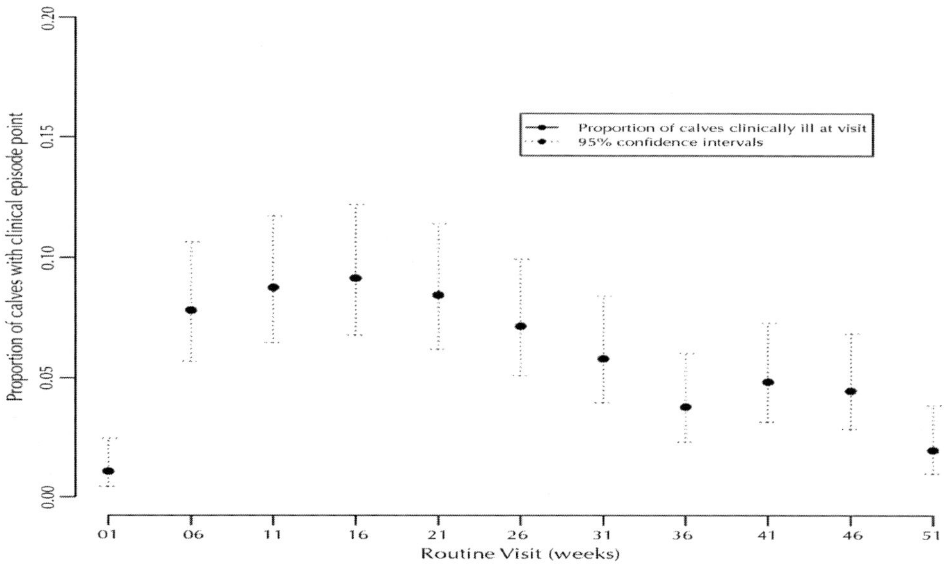

Figure 7: The distribution of the proportion of calves classed as having a clinical episode stratified by visit number over the 51 weeks of observations for each calf in the IDEAL project.

Pathogens and Exposures

Figure 8 shows the list of pathogen/test combinations experienced by the calf by the time of publication crudely stratified into endoparasites, haemoparasites, bacteria and viruses. Some of the common pathogens such as *Theileria spp.* appear several times as a number of techniques were used to identify them. In addition, some assays, such as microscopy, do not distinguish between species. More detailed analysis of these co-infections is ongoing. What this Figure shows very clearly is that this population of calves is infected with over 50 different pathogens and has been exposed to at least a further 6 bacteria and viruses. However, relatively few pathogens were found in the majority of calves, and the main pathogens were helminths and protozoan haemoparasites. What is of particular interest is that, given such high incidences of these key pathogens such as *T. parva*, *A. marginale*, *B. bigemina* and *H. placei*, why more of these calves did not die. One of the main objectives of the continuing analyses of this dataset is to unravel the coinfections and relate these to the calf genotype and key outcomes such as growth rate, morbidity and mortality. It is also interesting that there are very few bacterial diagnoses and these appear to have only sporadic occurrence and rarely contributed to death. We plan to look in more detail at the dam serology, but of the 2 bacterial pathogen exposures already measured in the dams, *Brucella spp.* and *Leptospira hardjo* the seroprevalences were extremely low, 0.036 (0.022-0.050 adjusted 95% CI) and 0.068 (0.035-0.101 95% adjusted CI) respectively. Also there was little clinical evidence of some of the major viral diseases such as foot-and-mouth disease.

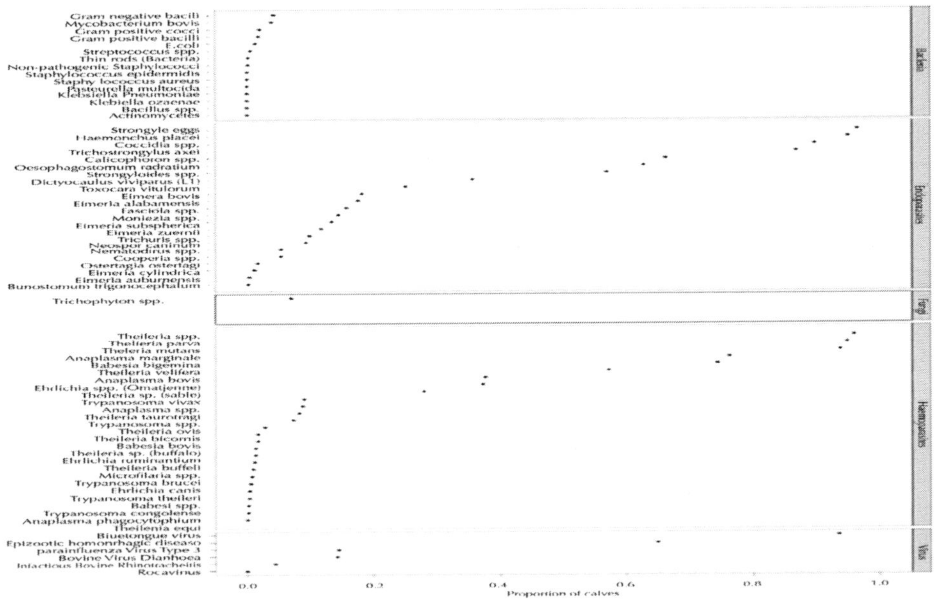

Figure 8: The proportion of animals positive for a given pathogen/test combination at any time through the course of the 51 weeks of observation on each calf in the IDEAL project.

DISCUSSION

The IDEAL project is the first attempt to describe the entire disease burden of any naturally occurring population. Funding was only available to follow calves for the first 12 months of life. The use of a longitudinal design, though enormously logistically challenging in this environment, allowed us to generate a unique dataset to study the effects of co-infections in the SHZ breed in this small holder setting.

This may be applicable across a large sector of the Great Lakes basin where very similar breeds and husbandry are in operation.

When designing the project a number of different approaches were considered. They included stratification by management system, wealth/herd size, livestock distribution, location, ethnicity, etc. However, the lack of available data on several of these factors led to the decision to stratify by agro-ecological zone only. Random cluster sampling will have ensured that reasonable representation was provided for the various levels of each of the un-stratified factors, i.e. the total sample size will include farmers with varying herd sizes and management systems. The proportion of sub-locations sampled in each AEZ is in proportion of each AEZ in the total survey area (based on numbers of sub-locations). The study was constrained by logistics to an area of 45 km radius from Busia town in order to make repeated visits possible. Initially other options were reviewed but following piloting of sampling in the field it became clear that given the road conditions and number of animals that would have to be sampled per day at the peak of sampling in year 2 this was the most practical approach.

Owners were paid a retainer for the year to allow access to the animals and therefore compliance was very high. There were a small number of instances of animals being stolen and of owners treating the calves with anthelminthics without consulting the project vet. Where these were identified animals were censored and their data from the visit following treatment discarded.

The descriptive analysis from the recruitment interview indicates that livestock production in this system is characterised by low-input, with as few as 30% of the farms carrying out any form of disease control during the follow-up time. Even for those farms that reported carrying out disease control measures, the frequency of these per year was below what would be effective. This level of management would likely be insufficient to support the use of improved "exotic" breeds which are kept in the region but which we intentionally excluded from this study. The Western Province of Kenya accounts for only 4% of Kenya's total exotic dairy herd [43]. This is despite major breed improvements programs instituted to support smallholder farmers in the region through increased livestock productivity [43,44].

Livestock disease and vector control are required for increased livestock productivity, and prevention of losses through disease-related morbidity, mortality, and loss of markets for livestock products. The observed lack of disease control has implications on some of the strategies envisaged to rapidly improve livestock-dependent livelihoods. It also highlights the need to provide support not just for the imported exotic breeds but also for the indigenous breeds in order to minimise the losses and maximise productivity. The consistent use of disease control practices has contributed to the relative success of the smallholder dairy sector in the Kenyan highlands [45]. The benefits of such controls, carried out at community level, have also been demonstrated in other settings [46]. Failure to consider these disease issues is recognised as a factor that could seriously reduce rural growth [47].

Many countries in sub-Saharan Africa have had to make structural adjustments to their veterinary infrastructure and the services they provide which leave farmers and herdsmen without the support needed to introduce exotic genetic stock. Further, Rege *et al.*[48] argue that breeding strategies in the context of smallholder farms should be based on improving food security, income and overall livelihoods of the livestock keepers and should not be based on genetic improvement of livestock. Focus should be on providing the most appropriate genotypes in a local context. However, identifying these appropriate genotypes is itself complex. Mwachara *et al.* [49] identify the need to involve the livestock keepers in designing the breeding programmes to take into account the full array of contributions to livelihoods that these animals make and so identify genetic characteristics related to these functions. Whereas most programs have concentrated on cross-breeding, there exists a lot of potential and advantages for improvements based on within-breed selection.

The mortality rates in this indigenous calf population were higher than anticipated at the design stage. There are few reports that we could find from similar systems but other reports from the region suggest a range of mortalities. Barnett [50] reported a mortality rate of 29% from a study based in Western Province Kenya. In a Tanzanian smallholder dairy system mortality rates of 35% were reported [51] within the first year with 42% reported as of unknown cause and 19% due to redwater (babesiosis). Swai *et al.*[52] reported mortality rates of 12% in small holder dairy systems in Zimbabwe with 56% ascribed to tick borne disease particularly east coast fever. Gitau *et al.*[53] reported 7% mortality in calves up to 6 months of age from the same area of Western. A more recent large study of calf mortality in Mali [54] reported an overall calf mortality of 17% but when this was broken down by system the more intensive systems had high mortality rates of 19% and 25% compared to 10% in the traditional pastoralist systems. Interestingly they report gastrointestinal disorders as causing 28% of their overall mortality followed by perinatal problems (16%) and accidents (14%). Direct comparisons are very difficult to make with many of these studies as the design; breeds, environment etc are not the same. However, it is useful to get an overall impression of how these animals are performing in this system. The mortality rate in the IDEAL cohort appears high given it is an indigenous breed that might be expected to have had time to adapt to the conditions. There are likely to be many contributing causes including possible inexperience in raising cattle compared to traditional cattle owning groups such as the Maasai or Fulani and the co-infection combinations present in the region.

The identification of pathogens at all-time points in the study is ongoing. We adopted a very pragmatic approach using the best field techniques available as the method of diagnosis but for many pathogens this is not sufficient. For example speciation of *Theileria* parasites requires more detailed analysis such as RLB [55]. It must be noted that detection of pathogens is limited by the sensitivity of the assay, the presence of the pathogen at the time of sampling and its location in the tissue which is sampled. This presents many challenges in trying to produce a definitive list of pathogens at every time point for each calf. For this preliminary presentation of the pathogens we have simply summed across all visits to estimate the proportion of calves with each pathogen (or pathogen/test combination). This ignores the dynamics of the order of exposure but this is to be reported in a number of other papers. The list of pathogens is extensive but there are actually only a few very high prevalence pathogens. These are mainly gut helminths and tick borne haemoparasites, in particular*T. parva*.

The IDEAL project provides unique data on total livestock disease burden in the region, which will allow for ranking of infectious diseases in order of importance. Such data are important for prioritising interventions, the absence of which up to this point has led to a lack of metrics to assess the impact of livestock diseases leads and therefore inefficient resource allocation [2]. In addition, the project will provide data on the within breed variation of key traits such as growth rates, clinical tolerance and resistance, and survival. This provides a basis for identifying desirable traits that may be taken up while designing within-breed improvement programs. Within-breed selection may not achieve increased productivity per animal as rapidly as cross-breeding methods, but offers the opportunity to retain the adaptive characteristics already present in indigenous breeds and which may offer opportunity for adaptation to changing climates. The findings of positive associations between knowledge of diseases and access to veterinary support with whether farmers carry out disease control practices supports the idea that increased extension services would have significant positive effect on livestock productivity.

CONCLUSIONS

This population of calves is the first to have a comprehensive investigation of the pathogen burden and exposures of any animal population. The analyses of the biobanked samples will continue and it is expected that there will be further pathogens added to the list. This preliminary report on the IDEAL project design and data collection offers an overview of the farming system in Western, Kenya, and of the infectious disease challenges experienced by the calves of the region. It provides a detailed description of the methods used to collect this detailed longitudinal dataset. This provides more information for those reading analytical papers from the project, and acts as a supporting document to the extensive biobank held at ILRI, Nairobi. It gives preliminary results and offers an overview of more detailed analyses that result from the IDEAL project.

AUTHORS' CONTRIBUTIONS

MW conceived the original idea and design and directed the project; MB was responsible for the study design, development of the clinical tools such as questionnaires, sample flows and diseases to be screened, data management and analysis and training of field staff; JP was responsible for the design and random sampling protocols, database management and data analysis; IH was responsible for management of the database, data extraction and analysis; HK was responsible for parasitology protocols and overall managing the project, the sample flows and diseases to be screened for and biobank management; PT was responsible for the management and interpretation of the serological screening of samples; KC was responsible for the clinical protocols, postmortem protocols, interpretation of clinical and postmortem data and training of the field staff; and OH and MN were responsible for managing the phenyotypic protocols and analysis and interpretation of the genetic data components. ST, IC and AJ were the veterinary surgeons in the field and as well as carrying out the clinical work and managing staff on the ground participated in the development of the tools and interpretation of the results. OT designed and implemented the database for the project and contributed to the design of the study. All authors read and approved the final manuscript.

ACKNOWLEDGEMENTS

The authors would like to thank the Wellcome Trust (grant No. 079445) for financial support for the project. We would like to thank the Kenyan Department of Veterinary Services for their enormous support in setting up the study and working with our teams in the field. We would also like to thank the many local animal health assistants and farmers who participated in the running of the project. Finally we would like to recognise the enormous contribution of Dr. Magai Kaare who worked as the IDEAL project manager until his untimely death following a car accident in 2008. He will be greatly missed by all who knew him.

REFERENCES

1. United Nations Department of Economic and Social Affairs Population Division: World population prospects: The 2008 revision, highlights, working paper no. ESA/P/WP,.2009. 210
2. Perry B, Grace D: The impacts of livestock diseases and their control on growth and development processes that are pro-poor. *Philos Trans R Soc Lond B Biol Sci* 2009, 364(1530):2643-2655.
3. Phiri BJ, Benschop J, French NP: Systematic review of causes and factors associated with morbidity and mortality on smallholder dairy farms in Eastern and Southern Africa. *Prev Vet Med* 2010, 94(1–2):1-8.

4. Perry BD, Rich KM: Poverty impacts of foot-and-mouth disease and the poverty reduction implications of its control. *Vet Rec* 2007, 160(7):238-+. [Times Cited: 0]

5. Morens DM, Holmes EC, Davis AS, Taubenberger JK: Global rinderpest eradication: lessons learned and why humans should celebrate too. *J Infect Dis* 2011, 204:502-505.

6. Zhang XS, Woolhouse MEJ: Escherichia coli O157 infection on Scottish cattle farms: dynamics and control. *J R Soc Interface* 2011, 8(60):1051-1058.

7. Bronsvoort B, Radford A, Tanya V, Kitching RP, Morgan K: The molecular epidemiology of foot-and-mouth disease viruses in the Adamawa Province of Cameroon. *J Clin Microbiol* 2004, 42(5):2186-2196

8. Gachohi JM, Kitala PM, Ngumi PN, Skilton RA: Environment and farm factors associated with exposure to Theileria parva infection in cattle under traditional mixed farming system in Mbeere District, Kenya. *Trop Anim Health Prod* 2011, 43:271-277.

9. Geiger SM: Immuno-epidemiology of Schistosoma mansoni infections in endemic populations co-infected with soil-transmitted helminths: Present knowledge, challenges, and the need for further studies. *Acta Tropica* 2008, 108(2–3):118-123.

10. Woolhouse M, Taylor L, Haydon D: Population biology of multihost pathogens. *Science* 2001, 292(5519):1109-1112.

11. Woolhouse M, Webster J, Domingo E, Charlesworth B, Levin B: Biological and biomedical implications of the co-evolution of pathogens and their hosts. *Nat Genet* 2002, 32(4):569-577.

12. Rohani P, Green C, Mantilla-Beniers N, Grenfell B: Ecological interference between fatal diseases. *Nature* 2003, 422(6934):885-888.

13. Morand S, Manning S, Woolhouse M: Parasite-host coevolution and geographic patterns of parasite infectivity and host susceptibility. *Proc R Soc London Ser B-Biol Sci* 1996, 263(1366):119-128.

14. Donoghue H, Marcsik A, Matheson C, Vernon K, Nuorala E, Molto J, Greenblatt C, Spigelman M:Co-infection of Mycobacterium tuberculosis and Mycobacterium leprae in human archaeological samples: a possible explanation for the historical decline of leprosy. *Proc R Soc B-Biol Sci* 2005, 272(1561):389-394.

15. Fall A, Diack A, Diaite A, Seye M, d'Ieteren G: Tsetse challenge, trypanosome and helminth infection in relation to productivity of village Ndama cattle in Senegal. *Vet Parasitol* 1999, 81(3):235-247.
16. Zinsstag J, Ankers P, Ndao M, Bonfoh B, Pfister K: Multiparasitism, production and economics in domestic animals in sub-Saharan West Africa. *Parasitol Today* 1998, 14(2):46-49.
17. Kaufmann J, Dwinger R, Hallebeek A, Vandijk B, Pfister K: The interaction of Trypanosoma congolense and Haemonchus contortus infections in trypanotolerant ndama 520 cattle. *Vet Parasitol* 1992, 43(3–4):157-170.
18. Flynn RJ, Mulcahy G, Welsh M, Cassidy JP, Corbett D, Milligan C, Andersen P, Strain S, McNair J:Co-Infection of cattle with Fasciola hepatica and Mycobacterium bovis - immunological consequences. *Transbound Emerg Dis* 2009, 56(6–7):269-274.
19. Carslake D, Grant W, Green LE, Cave J, Greaves J, Keeling M, McEldowney J, Weldegebriel H, Medley GF: Endemic cattle diseases: comparative epidemiology and governance. *Philos Trans R Soc Lond B Biol Sci* 2011, 366(1573):1975-1986.
20. Rafi W, Ribeiro-Rodrigues R, Ellner JJ, Salgame P: 'Coinfection-helminthes and tuberculosis'. *Curr Opin HIV AIDS* 2012, 7(3):239-244.
21. Cooper P, Chico M, Losonsky G, Sandoval C, Espinel I, Sridhara R, Aguilar M, Guevara A, Guderian R, Levine M, Griffin G, Nutman T: Albendazole treatment of children with ascariasis enhances the vibriocidal antibody response to the live attenuated oral cholera vaccine CVD 103-HgR. *J Infect Dis* 2000, 182(4):1199-1206.
22. Yazdanbakhsh M, Kremsner P, van Ree R: Immunology - Allergy, parasites, and the hygiene hypothesis. *Science* 2002, 296(5567):490-494.
23. Cleaveland S, Laurenson MK, Taylor LH: Diseases of humans and their domestic mammals: pathogen characteristics, host range and the risk of emergence. *Philos Trans R Soc Lond B Biol Sci* 2001, 356(1411):991-999.
24. Hanotte O, Dessie T, Kemp S: Time to tap Africa's livestock genomes. *Science* 2010, 328(5986):1640-1641.

25. Claridge J, Diggle P, McCann CM, Mulcahy G, Flynn R, McNair J, Strain S, Welsh M, Baylis M, Williams DJ: Fasciola hepatica is associated with the failure to detect bovine tuberculosis in dairy cattle. *Nat Commun* 2012, 3(5):853.
26. Zinsstag J, Schelling E, Roth F, Bonfoh B, de Savigny D, Tanner M: Human benefits of animal interventions for zoonosis control. *Emerg Infect Dis* 2007, 13(4):527-531.
27. Jaeztold R, Schmidt H: *Farm Management Handbook of Kenya, Part IIA, West Kenya. Nyanza and Western Provinces*. Kenya: Kenyan Ministry of Agriculture; 1983. p.387
28. Thornton P, Kruska R, Henninger N, Kristjanson P, Reid R, Atieno F, Odero A, Ndegwa T:*Mapping Poverty and Livestock in the Developing World. ILRI (International Livestock Research Institute)*. Nairobi: ILRI; 2002.
29. GOK: *Geographical Dimensions of Well-Being in Kenya. Where the Poor Live. Ministry of Planning and National Development*. Nairobi: Regal Press; 2003.
30. IFAD: *Assessment of Rural Poverty: Eastern and Southern Africa*. Rome: International Fund for Agricultural Development; 2002.
31. Reynecke DP, Van Wyk Ja, Gummow B, Dorny P, Boomker J: Application of ROC curve analysis to FAMACHA(©) evaluation of haemonchosis on two sheep farms in South. *Vet Parasitol* 2011, 177(3–4):224-230.
32. Gubbels JM, De Vos AP, Van der Weide M, Viseras J, Schouls LM, De Vries E, Jongejan F:Simultaneous detection of bovine Theileria and Babesia species by reverse line blot hybridization. *J Clin Microbiol* 1999, 37(6):1782-1789.
33. Taylor MA, Coop RL, Wall R: *Veterinary Parasitology*. Oxford, UK: Blackwell Publishing Ltd; 2007. ISBN 1405119640
34. Renz A, Trees AJ, Achukwi D, Edwards G, Wahl G: Evaluation of Suramin, Ivermectin and Cgp-20376 in a New Macrofilaricidal drug screen, Onchocerca-Ochengi in African cattle. *Trop Med Parasitol* 1995, 46:31-37. [QQ463 TROP MED PARASITOL]
35. Nicholson M, Butterworth M: *A Guide to Condition Scoring of Zebu Cattle*. Addis Ababa: International Livestock Centre for Africa; 1986.

36. OW Schalm DN: Experiments and observations leading to development of the California mastitis test. *J Am Vet Med Assoc* 1957, 130:199-204.
37. Jahnke HE: *Livestock Production Systems and Livestock Development in Tropical Africa*. Kiel: Kieler Wissenschaftsverlag Vauk; 1982.
38. ILCA: Handbook of African livestock statistics. Tech. rep., Addis Ababa: International Livestock Centre for Africa; 1993
39. Njuki J, Poole N, Johnson J, Baltenweck I, Pali P: Gender, livestock and livelihood indicators. Tech. rep., International Livestock Research Institute (ILRI) 2011.http://results.waterandfood.org/handle/10568/3036.
40. Kaplan EL, Meier P: Nonparametric estimation from incomplete observations. *J Am Stat Assoc* 1958, 53(282):457-481.
41. Kristjanson P, Krishna A, Radeny M, Nindo W: *Pathways out of Poverty in Western Kenya and the Role of Livestock*. FAO; 2004. http://hdl.handle.net/10568/1212.
42. Zaibet L, Traore S, Ayantunde A, Marshall K, Johnson N, Siegmund-Schultze M: Livelihood strategies in endemic livestock production systems in sub-humid zone of West Africa: trends, trade-offs and implications. *Env Dev Sustainability* 2011, 13:87-105.
43. Mudavadi PO, Otieno K, Wanambacha JW, Odenya JO: Smallholder dairy production and marketing in Western Kenya: a review of literature. Tech. rep., MOARD/KARI/ILRI 2001.http://hdl.handle.net/10568/1781.
44. Waithaka M, Nyangaga J, Staal S, Wokabi A, Njubi D, Muriuki K, Njoroge L, Wanjohi P:Characterization of dairy systems in the western Kenya region. Tech. rep., Smallholder Dairy (R&D) Project MALDM-KARI-ILRI-DFID, Nairobi, Kenya 2002.http://dspacetest.cgiar.org/handle/10568/1859
45. Omore A, Muriuki H, Kenyanjui M, Owango M, Staal S: The Kenya dairy sub-sector: a rapid appraisal. Tech. rep., ILRI 1999. http://dspacetest.cgiar.org/handle/10568/2054.
46. Hüttner K: The effect of a community-based animal health service programme on livestock mortality, off-take and selected husbandry applications A field study in northern Malawi. *Livest Prod Sci* 2001, 72(3):263-278. http://linkinghub.elsevier.com/retrieve/pii/S0301622601001877.

47. FAO: The state of food and agriculture, livestock in the balance. Rome, 2009. ISBN 9789251062159

48. Rege J, Marshall K, Notenbaert A, Ojango J, Okeyo A: Pro-poor animal improvement and breeding — What can science do? *Livest Sci* 2011, 136:15-28. http://linkinghub.elsevier.com/retrieve/pii/S1871141310004774

49. Mwacharo JM, Drucker AG: Production objectives and management strategies of livestock keepers in South-East Kenya: implications for a breeding programme. *Trop Anim Health Prod* 2005, 37(8):635-652. http://www.springerlink.com/index/10.1007/s11250-005-4253-8

50. Barnett S: Theileriasis control. *Bull Epiz Dis Afr* 1957, 5:343-357.

51. French N, Tyrer J, Hirst W: Smallholder dairy farming in the Chikwaka communal land, Zimbabwe: birth, death and demographic trends. *Prev Vet Med* 2001, 48:101-112.

52. Swai E, Karimuribo ED, Kambarage DM, Moshy WE: A longitudinal study on morbidity and mortality in youngstock smallholder dairy cattle with special reference to tick borne infections in Tanga region, Tanzania. *Vet Parasitol* 2009, 160:34-42.

53. Gitau G, Perry B, McDermott J: The incidence, calf morbidity and mortality due to Theileria parva infections in smallholder dairy farms in Murang'a District, Kenya. *Prev Vet Med* 1999, 39:65-79.

54. Wymann MN, Bonfoh B, Schelling E, Bengaly S, Tembely S, Tanner M, Zinsstag J: Calf mortality rate and causes of death under different herd management systems in peri-urban Bamako, Mali. *Livest Sci* 2006, 100:169-178.

55. Oura CAL, Bishop RP, Wampande EM, Lubega GW, Tait A: Application of a reverse line blot assay to the study of haemoparasites in cattle in Uganda. *Int J Parasitol* 2004, 34(5):603-613. [815TG INT J PARASITOL]

Chapter 5

Concepts for Risk-Based Surveillance in the Field of Veterinary Medicine and Veterinary Public Health: Review of Current Approaches

Katharina DC Stärk[1], Gertraud Regula[1], Jorge Hernandez[2], Lea Knopf[1], Klemens Fuchs[3], Roger S Morris[4], and Peter Davies[5]

[1]Federal Veterinary Office, CH-3003 Bern, Switzerland

[2]College of Veterinary Medicine, University of Florida, Gainsville, FL, USA

[3]Institute of Applied Statistics, A-8010 Graz, Austria

[4]EpiCentre, Massey University, Palmerston North, New Zealand

[5]Department of Veterinary Population Medicine, St. Paul, MN 55108, USA

ABSTRACT

Background

Emerging animal and zoonotic diseases and increasing international trade have resulted in an increased demand for veterinary surveillance systems. However, human and financial resources available to support government veterinary services are becoming more and more limited in many countries world-wide. Intuitively, issues that present higher risks merit higher priority for surveillance resources as investments will yield higher benefit-cost ratios. The rapid rate of acceptance of this core concept of risk-based surveillance has outpaced the development of its theoretical and practical bases.

Discussion

The principal objectives of risk-based veterinary surveillance are to identify surveillance needs to protect the health of livestock and consumers, to set priorities, and to allocate resources effectively and efficiently. An important goal is to achieve a higher benefit-cost ratio with existing or reduced resources. We propose to define risk-based surveillance systems as those that apply risk assessment methods in different steps of traditional surveillance design for early detection and management of diseases or hazards. In risk-based designs, public health, economic and trade consequences of diseases play an important role in selection of diseases or hazards. Furthermore, certain strata of the population of interest have a higher probability to be sampled for detection of diseases or hazards. Evaluation of risk-based surveillance systems shall prove that the efficacy of risk-based systems is equal or higher than traditional systems; however, the efficiency (benefit-cost ratio) shall be higher in risk-based surveillance systems.

Summary

Risk-based surveillance considerations are useful to support both strategic and operational decision making. This article highlights applications of risk-based surveillance systems in the veterinary field including food safety. Examples are provided for risk-based hazard selection, risk-based selection of sampling strata as well as sample size calculation based on risk considerations.

BACKGROUND

Emerging animal and zoonotic diseases and increasing international trade have resulted in an increased demand for veterinary surveillance systems, while human and financial resources available to support government veterinary services are becoming more and more limited in many countries world-wide. This constrains all areas of activities of veterinary services, including monitoring and surveillance programmes. One option to respond to this situation is to ensure that the most relevant programmes are maintained. Several government veterinary services, including those of England and Wales (Anonymous, 2000) and New Zealand (Thornton, 2004) have therefore undertaken evaluations of their surveillance programmes. One recommendation of the review in England and Wales was that a structured approach was needed to determine priorities for surveillance, and that this approach should be based on risk (Anonymous, 2000). Consequently, a method to develop risk profiles for animal diseases is being developed (Anonymous, 2003). A similar outcome resulted from the evaluation of surveillance needs in New Zealand, which stated that a 'risk-based' approach to identify priority diseases will provide the basis for resource allocation (Thornton, 2004). These examples illustrate the background and motivation behind the 'risk-based' philosophy for veterinary surveillance. The core rationale underpinning risk-based strategies is that issues that present higher risks merit higher priority for surveillance resources as these investments will yield higher benefit-cost ratios. This axiomatic foundation has led to a rapid rate of acceptance of the concept of risk-based surveillance that has outpaced the development of its theoretical and practical bases. The phrase 'risk-based surveillance' is increasingly prevalent in government documents of many countries, being applied across a range of contexts including chemical residue monitoring, exotic disease surveillance, or sampling for food safety assurance in general.

Inevitably, because the term 'risk' is defined differently in various contexts, its use in relation to surveillance has tended to be vague.

The objectives of this article are to review reports on risk-based surveillance, and to develop a framework which may hopefully lead to more uniform use and understanding of both the terminology and its practical implementation.

REVIEW AND DISCUSSION

Terminology

In order to discuss 'risk-based' surveillance, it is essential to clarify the meaning of risk. Risk (as a noun) has numerous common language uses that influence its interpretation. A short list includes 1) the chance of something going wrong; 2) any hazardous entity likely to cause injury, damage, or loss; 3) in insurance, the probability, amount, or type of possible loss incurred and covered by an insurer; 4) in finance, the possibility of loss in an investment or speculation.

Risk has been defined by medical epidemiologists as 'the probability of disease developing in an individual in a specified time interval' (Rothman and Greenland, 1998). In contrast, in the field of risk analysis, risk is defined as the synthesis of two components, namely the probability of occurrence of an undesired event and the consequences or costs of this event (International Animal Health Code). The Society for Risk Analysis defines risk as 'the potential for realization of unwanted, adverse consequences to human life, health, property, or the environment; estimation of risk is usually based on the expected value of the probability of the event occurring times the consequence of the event given that it has occurred.' Thus risk may be viewed as the absolute value of expected losses. We would argue that the epidemiological definition for risk (probability only) is less useful in the context of surveillance than the risk analysis paradigm, because the probability of occurrence of an adverse event alone is not sufficient to drive allocation of resources, and expected consequences of disease events must have substantial influence.

Furthermore, risk is being evaluated in the framework of risk analysis consisting of risk management, risk assessment and risk communication (International Animal Health Code). Surveillance itself is an integral component of both risk management (e.g., as a tool for early detection of an event) and risk communication. The term 'risk-based surveillance' could consequently imply that allocation of surveillance activities is guided by the probability of events with or without consideration of the consequences of the event; the management of the event; or the process of communication (including perceptions) of the event.

The term 'targeted' surveillance has been used to describe concepts which, from an epidemiological perspective, could constitute risk-based surveillance. This term was first used with reference to surveillance programmes of bovine spongiform encephalopathy (BSE) (Doherr et al., 2001, 2002; Morignat et al., 2002). The concept of targeted surveillance for BSE was to concentrate sampling for screening tests on defined sub-populations of cattle that were expected to have a higher prevalence of the disease (Doherr et al., 2001). The sub-populations were defined by age and by so-called 'exit routes', i.e. whether cattle went to normal slaughter, emergency slaughter or were cattle that died or were euthanised at the farm. Similarly, targeted surveillance was defined more generally as surveillance 'focusing the sampling on high-risk populations in which specific, commonly known risk factors exist' under the assumption that the event to be surveyed would be more common in the targeted population than in the general population (Salman et al., 2003). Assuming that the epidemiological intelligence is correct (i.e. high-risk groups can be predicted from risk factors), for a fixed surveillance investment, targeted surveillance should yield both higher sensitivity and higher positive predictive value than surveillance conducted randomly across the population. Martin and Cameron (2003) argue that the assumption in traditional surveillance, that the probability of disease is constant across all individuals in the reference population is not realistic. They propose the evaluation of surveillance systems using scenario trees. The nodes of their trees represent factors affecting the probability of disease occurrence in sub-populations that may be targeted by surveillance. Elsewhere, targeted surveillance was defined as surveillance "to answer a specific question about a defined disease or condition using agreed mechanisms for detection" (Anonymous, 2003), a definition which does not explicitly incorporate risk-based concepts.

In the context of food safety, a 'risk-based food safety system' has been defined by the SaFoodChain working group (SaFoodChain website). This definition states that a risk-based food safety system is 'a system that demonstrates to consumers and other stakeholders that foods are being produced under conditions which minimize adverse health effects. This is achieved by using information on the nature of human health hazards associated with particular food products, the likelihood of consumers being exposed to these hazards, the consequences of exposure and the capacity of the production and processing system to mitigate risks arising from hazards which are above a threshold of concern'. The motivation behind this approach is to promote efficient risk management and to facilitate risk communication, primarily in the context of quality assurance.

Risk-Based Approaches in Disciplines other than Veterinary Medicine

Risk-based approaches are widely used in many fields unrelated to animal health. Particularly, ecologists have widely adopted risk-based methods. In the management of environmental pollution risks, the so-called 'risk-based corrective action' (RBCA, 'Rebecca') has become a standard (Standard guide for risk-based corrective action). The formal definition of RBCA is: "A streamlined approach in which exposure and risk assessment practices are integrated with traditional components of the corrective action process to ensure that appropriate and cost-effective remedies are selected, and that limited resources are properly allocated" (EPA, 1995). In RBCA, contaminated sites are classified (scored) according to exposure scenarios and consequences to public health. Corrective actions are then defined for the different site categories. In the categorisation, four tiers of risk assessment were described where the level of detail and complexity of the risk assessment increases from tier I to tier IV ("Use of risk-based decision making").

Modelling approaches have also been used in environmental sciences to predict likely sites of contamination or spills with the objective to target intervention and to obtain cost-effective surveillance (Smalley et al., 2000) or for early warning purposes (Grayman and Males, 2002). Furthermore, environmental scientists developed sampling methods that take into account risk factors for contamination, specifically in water. Such risk-based sampling has been described for heavy metals in water (Preston and Shackelford, 2002), and for watershed monitoring (Foran et al., 2000). Risk-based sampling was also applied using spatial risk factors (Ericson and Gonzalez, 2003).

In the management of both private and government businesses, risk-based auditing is a broadly known concept. This method is primarily used for internal auditing and qualitative scores are used to categorise activities with respect to business risks (McNamee, 1997). Managers are expected to monitor their management practices and processes with special focus on major business risks, e.g. market or financial risks. The motivation for this approach appears to be similar to the motivation behind risk-based surveillance, namely: "The identification, prioritization and sourcing of key organizational risks is critical to ensuring that internal audit resources are allocated to the areas that matter most". Risk-based auditing was also described with relation to auditing of research grants and auditing of subsidy payments.

Closer to the veterinary field, risk-based concepts are applied in the surveillance of human diseases. In Italy, special surveillance programmes were implemented for workers who are exposed to specific occupational risks (Franco et al., 2002). The risk categorisation of workers in this example included both scientific evidence as well as risk perception. The objective of this approach was early detection of disease. Similar concepts are applied in screening programmes focusing on certain age groups, e.g. mammography in women or prostate cancer in men.

Proposed Concepts

In animal health surveillance, decisions at operational or strategic levels can be distinguished. Strategic decisions are needed regarding which issues warrant surveillance, and operational decisions assure the most effective use of resources based on epidemiological principles. One possible framework for terminology, in line with previous authors (Doherr et a., 2001, 2002; Morignat et al., 2002; Salman et al. 2003), would be for the term 'targeted surveillance' to denote use of epidemiological risk factors to optimize population sampling at an operational level. The term 'risk-based surveillance' could be reserved for the context of strategic decision making that employs principles of risk analysis in relation to surveillance of animal disease.

An alternative, that we recommend, is that risk-based surveillance be defined as a more inclusive term in which both the epidemiological and risk analysis perspectives are integrated. Based on the definition of risk and the review of the use of the term 'risk-based' in various fields, we propose to define risk-based veterinary surveillance as follows:

A surveillance programme in the design of which exposure and risk assessment methods have been applied together with traditional design approaches in order to assure appropriate and cost-effective data collection.

This relatively broad definition allows for the application of risk assessment approaches at all steps of the design of surveillance systems for early detection and management of diseases or hazards of interest. Table 1 illustrates the different steps during design where surveillance can be based on risk assessment principles. These options for risk-based design will be illustrated in the later sections of this article.

Table 1: Steps in the design of veterinary or food safety surveillance programmes, the possible application of risk assessment steps to obtain risk-based surveillance programmes and the epidemiological contributions providing the basis for risk assessments

Surveillance design steps	Risk assessment steps	Epidemiological contributions	Examples	References
Selection of disease or agent	Hazard identification, hazard characterisation, exposure assessment, consequence assessment	Case reporting, outbreak investigations, systematic review	Selection of diseases based on economic significance for producers, selection of zoonotic agents based on public health significance	Paige et al., 1999; Stärk et al., 2000; Breidenbach et al., 2004; Brülisauer et al., 2004
Sampling				
Selection of strata	Exposure assessment, consequence assessment, risk factors	Risk factor studies, models for population attributable risk, meta analyses	Age strata, spatial strata (regions), product types, products from certain producers	Doherr et al., 2001; Morignat et al., 2002; Breidenbach et al., 2004; Brülisauer et al., 2004

Selection of units	Not applicable (random selection)			
Sample size	Release assessment	Random non-risk-based surveys, cross-sectional studies	Repeated surveys, confidence in disease freedom after defined time periods	Hadorn et al., 2002a

Stärk *et al. BMC Health Services Research* 2006 6:20 doi:10.1186/1472-6963-6-20

Considering the existing applications of risk-based veterinary surveillance programmes together with applications of risk-based methods in other fields, the objectives of the risk-based approach can be derived. The principal objectives of risk-based veterinary surveillance are:

- to identify surveillance needs to protect the health of livestock and consumers
- to set priorities,
- to allocate resources effectively and efficiently. An important goal is to achieve a higher benefit-cost ratio with existing or reduced resources.

In risk-based systems, public health, economic, and trade consequences of diseases play an important role in selection of diseases or hazards. Evaluation of risk-based surveillance systems shall prove that the efficacy of the risk-based approach is equal or higher than that of traditional surveillance; however, the efficiency (cost-benefit) shall be higher in risk-based systems.

The design of risk-based surveillance systems requires prior, epidemiological knowledge on, e.g., the difference in occurrence of disease between population strata or the influence of risk factors. This type of information cannot be generated by risk-based surveillance systems themselves, but needs to be obtained using traditional, quantitative epidemiological approaches (Table 1).

Risk-Based Hazard Selection

When surveillance programmes have broad objectives, the list of candidate hazards to be considered can be extensive and selection of hazards becomes critical. For example, the European Union requests that trading partners conduct monitoring of zoonotic pathogens in milk and milk products (Directive 92/46/EEC). The lists of different milk products on the market and potential hazards are very long. However, some agents cannot survive the processing steps employed for specific milk products. For example, Brülisauer et al. (2004) showed that surveillance of zoonotic bacteria in hard cheeses was not cost-effective because the probability of survival of these pathogens through the production process was extremely small. Other surveillance objectives with extensive lists of hazards include surveillance for chemical residues in animal-derived food and the monitoring of antimicrobial resistance in bacteria of animal origin. In both instances, risk-based hazard selection will be required to assure the most important hazards are included. Paige et al. (1999) described how risk profiles were used for substance selection in the national residue monitoring programme in the U.S.A. Ledergerber (2005) used risk profiling and risk ranking to prioritise combinations of bacteria and antimicrobial resistance which should be included in a classification scheme to identify livestock herds that harbour 'important' antimicrobial resistance patterns. For example, fluoroquinolone resistance in Salmonella and cephalosporine resistance in*E. coli* were ranked higher than ampicilline resistance in *E. coli* or Salmonella. This ranking was based on estimated health implications of these resistance patterns when transferred to humans.

The identification and selection of hazards are key steps in the design of surveillance systems, and they will be guided by the objectives of the surveillance. In risk assessment, the equivalent steps are hazard identification and hazard characterisation (Table 1). Consequences of hazard exposure should also be included in the characterisation of a hazard. A limitation in this respect is the lack of information on the nature and size of consequences. In the review of surveillance programmes in England and Wales, it was recommended to use a structured and transparent approach for hazard selection (Anonymous, 2000). Hazard selection was previously conducted with help of decision trees or flow charts in the context of serological surveillance programmes for exotic diseases in pigs in Denmark and Switzerland (Stärk et al., 2000;

Hadorn et al., 2002b). The proposed decision tree included hazard characteristics such as prevalence, performance of diagnostic tests, domestic economic implications and international trade implications. Epidemiological data on case frequencies due to specific hazards and results of outbreak investigations provide important input to the hazard identification step.

Risk-Based Selection of Population Strata

Once it has been decided which hazards should be included in a surveillance programme, the next step is the sampling design. In non-risk-based random sampling, all units in a population have the same probability to be selected (Cameron et al., 2003). Limitations of this approach have been identified by several authors. Key concerns are the economic viability of such surveillance programmes when the prevalence of the hazard approaches zero (Paisley, 2001; Doherr and Audigé, 2001; Webb et al., 2001). The cornerstone of risk-based sampling strategies is stratification of the target population into categories that display heterogeneity in probability of harbouring a hazard, or heterogeneity in the severity of consequence if the hazard is present. The probability of individual units within strata to be sampled can nevertheless be calculated, which makes this type of sampling a special case of probability sampling and different from non-probability or purposive sampling as described by Cameron et al. (2003). Strata to be used for risk-based sampling are derived from epidemiological studies assessing the probability of occurrence of the hazard in the stratum (e.g. herds having imported animals from abroad, herds with specific risk factors) and/or the consequence of the occurrence of the hazard in this stratum (e.g. potentially infected animals in sale yards or markets). Prior information on the probability of hazard occurrence in strata may originate from a range of quantitative epidemiological studies, e.g., risk factor studies. The risk of a stratum as part of a risk-based surveillance design can be derived qualitatively (a risk score or risk category) or quantitatively using risk assessment methods. Results of meta analyses can support this step. Similar to this approach, Thurmond (2003) described a sampling strategy referred to as "proportional risk sampling". In proportional risk sampling, the sample size in different strata reflects the respective risk level.

Unit selection within a risk stratum is done at random and all aspects of random sampling are applicable (Cameron et al., 2003). Issues to be considered in non-risk-based sampling such as test performance and clustering (Martin et al., 1992; Cameron and Baldock, 1998a and 1998b, Ziller et al., 2002) are equally relevant in risk-based sampling.

Many sampling schemes in surveillance programmes that use – at first sight – non-risk-based designs, turn out to use some kind of risk-based strata. For example, samples for laboratory testing are often collected from specified age groups of animals. The reason for this lies in the epidemiology of infectious diseases in populations. For example, older animals are more likely to have antibodies against a hazard (and therefore, to show positive serological results) because they were exposed to a hazard – if it was present. This makes this age group a 'high-probability' group according to our definition. More explicit stratum definitions can be found in protocols for BSE surveillance (see above; Doherr et al., 2001; Morignat et al., 2002).

A more complex approach to stratum definition which takes probability and public health consequence into account to monitor foreign substance levels in imported food of animal origin was described by Breidenbach et al. (2004). They developed a qualitative risk scoring system that took into account the residue legislation and surveillance programmes in the country of origin, the history of residue detection in commodities of the country of origin, the type of commodity (i.e. risk of accumulation of substances), and the public health significance of a substance. Combining these factors, a cumulative, relative risk score was calculated and all substance-commodity-country combinations with the highest scores were included in the programme.

Another way to define risk strata is the incorporation of spatial information. If the underlying phenomena show spatial dependency, point pattern analysis (Diggle, 1983), lattice data (Besage, 1974) or geostatistical methodology (Cressie, 1991) can be used to identify spatial risk factors. Fuchs et al. (2004) applied spatial point pattern analysis to study the resistance behaviour of*Enterococcus* to tetracycline in bulk milk and to identify high density and low density areas. To evaluate space-time interaction of scabies in Styrian chamois, Fuchs and Deutz (2002) used geostatistical methods to find critical distances. Wagner and Fuchs (2005) designed a risk-based sampling plan on the basis of spatial logistic regression for the BHV-1 monitoring in a free region.

Risk-Based Sample Size Calculation

If repeated surveys to document disease freedom are conducted, risk assessment methods can be useful to estimate the likely change in the probability of disease presence since the past survey. In using a risk-based approach, the sample size calculation takes into account the level of confidence that remains from previous survey. The necessary sample size for an upcoming survey is estimated based on the difference to the targeted level of confidence. This approach was proposed by Cannon (2001) and was applied in the context of surveillance to demonstrate freedom from disease by Hadorn et al. (2002a). In this application, a risk assessment was conducted to estimate the probability of hazard introduction (e.g. enzootic bovine leucosis) during a one-year period between two consecutive surveys. Introduction pathways considered were importation of live animals, migratory wildlife or vectors. It was shown that the required sample size for consecutive surveys could be reduced by 60–80 % (Hadorn et al., 2002a, Hadorn et al., 2002b). This reduction in sample size was primarily due to a limited number of live animals being imported from countries with a lower disease status. The accuracy of the estimated sample size does, however, depend on the completeness of the risk assessment. The latter should not only include the probability of hazard introduction but also the consequences of residual, non-detected infection in the country. Additionally, the "aging" of information originating from passed surveys needs to be considered. An improved risk model is being developed to address these issues (Knopf, personal communication).

Analysis and Integration of Data from Risk-Based Surveys

Data from risk-based surveillance can be analysed using similar analytical techniques as in non-risk-based surveys (see, for example, Dargatz and Hill, 1996; Audigé and Beckett, 1999; Suess et al., 2002), provided that risk assessment approaches are applied to hazard selection only and extrapolation of results to other hazards is not required. However, when population strata have been selected for sampling based on risk considerations, extrapolation of results to the general population is not possible unless the risk difference between high-risk and low-risk strata is known. This, however, may not be easy to assess. Martin and Cameron (2003) propose the use of scenario trees to compare the sensitivity of random surveillance systems with systems conducted in high-disease-probability populations. They define the *sensitivity ratio* as a measure to assess representativeness *vs*. the level of targeting in a surveillance system.

Furthermore, in international trade, the question of equivalence between sampling designs may become an issue. Trade between countries of equivalent animal health status does not pose a problem, but participating countries need to document their health status. However, when one country is using risk-based sampling and the other is not, they may operate surveillance systems at different confidence levels of case detection. If risk-based surveillance works as expected, a country using the risk-based approach should be more likely to detect positive samples than if using non-risk-based surveillance. This may lead to trade restrictions and other negative consequences. How can the results of one system be compared with the other? If this problem is not resolved, it is likely to pose a major barrier to the adoption of risk-based surveillance in relation to trade.

Another important issue is the integration of data from different sources, risk-based and non-risk-based. Although Cannon (2001) proposed an approach for use of data from different sources, data from risk-based surveillance designs were not considered. One data source may be historical data. The issue of weighting of historic data and the quantification of aging of data are unresolved (Thurmond, 2003). Graphical methods have also been proposed to integrate data from different sources (Hueston and Yoe, 2000), but reports of successful applications of this approach are lacking. In the context of BSE surveillance, where data is being collected from different risk-based population strata, the need of integration of surveillance results became evident (Ducrot et al., 2003).

SUMMARY

The need for efficient and cost-effective surveillance systems will induce the use of risk-based selection of hazards and population strata, and risk-based sample size calculation. Risk-based surveillance systems offer a more efficient approach for early detection and management of diseases. However, these innovative methods can only be established if there is international agreement on the methodology for risk-based surveillance, and the interpretation of its results. There is an urgent need for the development and evaluation of standardised, internationally accepted methods for risk-based surveillance.

AUTHORS' CONTRIBUTIONS

KS, GR, RM and LK developed the proposed concepts for risk-based surveillance. KS and PD were involved in drafting the article. KF contributed aspects on spatial risk. All authors read, critically revised and approved the final manuscript.

ACKNOWLEDGEMENTS

We thank all members of the SaFoodChain group for valuable discussions on risk-based approaches to food safety.

REFERENCES

1. Anoymous: Veterinary surveillance in England and Wales: A review. In *Report*. Ministry of Agriculture, Fisheries and Food, London; 2000.
2. Anoymous: Partnership, priorities and professionalism: A strategy for enhancing veterinary surveillance in the UK. In *Report*. Department for Environment, Food and Rural Affairs, London; 2003.
3. Audigé L, Beckett S: A quantitative assessment of the validity of animal-health surveys using stochastic modelling. *Prev Vet Med* 1999, 38:259-276.
4. Besage JE: Spatial interaction and the spatial analysis of lattice systems. *Journal of the Royal Statistical Society B* 1974, 36:192-225.
5. Breidenbach E, Sievi M, Weber U, Heiz H, Stärk KDC: Fundamental principles for risk-based planning of random sampling to trace hazard in imported meat. v*Proceedings 5th World Congress*

Foodborne Infections and Intoxications; 7 – 11 June 2004; Berlin 2004, in press.

6. Brülisauer F, Berger T, Klein B, Danuser J: Risk based surveillance of milk and dairy products. *Proceedings International ConferenceVeterinary Public Health and Food Safety – Towards a Risk based Chain Control: 22–23 October 2004; Rome. Istituto Zooprofilattico Sperimentale delle Regioni Lazio e Toscana* 2004, 50-51.
7. Cameron AR, Baldock FC: Two-stage sampling in surveys to substantiate freedom from disease. *Prev Vet Med* 1998, 34:19-30.
8. Cameron AR, Baldock FC: A new probability formula for surveys to substantiate freedom from disease. *Prev Vet Med* 1998, 34:1-17.
9. Cameron A, Gardner I, Doherr MG, Wagner B: Sampling considerations in surveys and monitoring and surveillance systems. In *Animal disease surveillance and survey systems – methods and applications*. Edited by Salman MD. Ames: Iowa State Press; 2003:47-66.
10. Cannon RM: Sense and sensitivity-designing surveys based on an imperfect test. *Prev Vet Med* 2001, 49:141-163.
11. Cressie NAC: *Statistics for Spatial Data*. New York, Chichester. Toronto: John Wiley & Sons; 1991.
12. Dargatz DA, Hill GW: Analysis of survey data. *Prev Vet Med* 1996, 28:225-237.
13. Diggle PJ: *Point pattern analysis*. London: Academic Press; 1983.
14. Doherr MG, Heim D, Fatzer R, Cohen CH, Vandevelde M, Zurbriggen A: Targeted screening of high-risk cattle populations for BSE to augment mandatory reporting of clinical suspects. *Prev Vet Med* 2001, 51:3-16.
15. Doherr MG, Hett AR, Cohen CH, Fatzer R, Rufenacht J, Zurbriggen A, Heim D: Trends in prevalence of BSE in Switzerland based on fallen stock and slaughter surveillance. *Vet Rec* 2002, 150:347-348.
16. Doherr MG, Audigé L: Monitoring and surveillance for rare health-related events: a review from the veterinary perspective. *Philos Trans R Soc Lond B Biol Sci* 2001, 356:1097-1106.

17. Ducrot C, Roy P, Morignat E, Baron T, Calavas D: How the surveillance system may bias the results of analytical epidemiological studies on BSE: prevalence among dairy versus beef suckler cattle breeds in France. *Vet Res* 2003, 32:185-192.
18. EPA: Use of risk-based decision-making in UST Corrective Action Programs. [http://www.epa.gov] *Report* U.S. Environmental Protection Agency, Office of Solid Waste and Emergency Response (OSWER) Directive 9610.17. Environmental Protection Agency; 1995.
19. Ericson JE, Gonzalez EJ: Hierarchical sampling of multiple strata: an innovative technique in exposure characterization. *Environ Res* 2003, 92:221-231.
20. Foran J, Brosnan T, Connor M, Delfino J, DePinto J, Dickson K, Humphrey H, Novotny V, Smith R, Sobsey M, Stehman S: A Framework for Comprehensive, Integrated, Watershed Monitoring in New York City. *Environ Monit Assess* 2000, 62:147-167.
21. Franco G, Cella MT, Tuccillo E, Ferrari F, Minisci E, Fusetti L: From risk-based health surveillance to health promotion: an evidence-based experience in a health care setting. *Int J Occup Med Environ Health* 2002, 15:117-120.
22. Fuchs K, Deutz A, Wagner P, Köfer J: Spatial point pattern analysis to study the resistance behaviour of enterococcus to tetracycline in bulk milk. In *Proceedings of the SVEPM: 24 – 26 March 2004*. Edited by Reid SWJ, Menzies FD, Russell AM. Martigny, Switzerland; 2004:134-142.
23. Fuchs K, Deutz A: Use of variograms to detect critical spatial distances for the Knox's test. *Prev Vet Med* 2002, 45:37-45.
24. Grayman WM, Males RM: Risk-based modeling of early warning systems for pollution accidents. *Water Sci Technol* 2002, 46:41-49.
25. Hadorn DC, Rüfenacht J, Hauser R, Stärk KDC: Risk-based design of repeated surveys for the documentation of freedom from non-highly contagious diseases. *Prev Vet Med* 2002, 56:179-192.
26. Hadorn DC, Hauser R, Stärk KDC: Epidemiologische Grundlagen und Resultate der Stichprobenuntersuchung 2001 in der schweizerischen Schweinepopulation. *Schweiz Arch Tierheilk* 2002, 144:532-541.

27. Hueston WD, Yoe CE: Estimating the overall power of complex surveillance systems.In *Proceedings of the 9th International Symposium on Veterinary Epidemiology and Economics: 6–11 August, 2000*. Edited by Salman MD, Morley PS, Ruch-Gallie R. Breckenridge, Colorado; 2000:758-760.

28. International Animal Health Code [http://www.oie.int] Office International des Epizooties, Paris;

29. Ledergerber U: Foundation of a herd classification scheme by risk profiling and risk ranking of antimicrobial resistance in the food chain. [http://www.dfvf.dk/Default.asp?ID=9726] *Report* International EpiLab, Copenhagen; 2005.

30. Martin SW, Shoukri M, Thorburn MA: Evaluating the health status of herds based on tests applied to individuals. *Prev Vet Med* 1992, 14:33-43.

31. Martin PAJ, Cameron A: Documenting freedom from avian influenza. In *Report*. International EpiLab, Copenhagen; 2003.

32. McNamee D: [http://www.mc2consulting.com] *Risk-based auditing for internal auditors*. Mc2 Management Consulting; 1997.

33. Morignat E, Ducrot C, Roy R, Baron T, Vinard JL, Biacabe AG, Madec JY, Bencsik A, Debeer S, Eliazsewicz M, Calavas D: Targeted surveillance to assess the prevalence of BSE in high-risk populations in western France and the associated risk factors. *Vet Rec* 2002, 151:73-77.

34. Paige JC, Chaudry MH, Pell FM: Federal surveillance of veterinary drugs and chemical residues (with recent data). *Veterinary Clinics of North America: Food Anim Pract* 1999, 15:45-60.

35. Paisley LG: Economic aspects of disease monitoring with special reference to bovine paratuberculosis. *Acta Vet Scand* 2001, (Suppl 94):17-25.

36. Preston BL, Shackelford J: Risk-Based Analysis of Environmental Monitoring Data: Application to Heavy Metals in North Carolina Surface Waters. *Environ Manage* 2002, 30:279-293.

37. Risk Analysis Glossary [http://www.sra.org/resources_glossary_p-r.php].

38. Rothman KJ, Greenland S: *Modern epidemiology*. 2nd edition. Philadelphia: Lippincott Williams & Wilkins; 1998.

39. SaFoodChain – the food safety consortium [http://www.safoodchain.org]
40. Salman MD, Stark KDC, Zepeda C: Quality assurance applied to animal disease surveillance systems. *Rev Sci Tech OIE* 2003, 22:689-696.
41. Smalley JB, Minsker BS, Goldberg DE: Risk-based in situ bioremediation design using a noisy genetic algorithm. *Water Ressour Res* 2000, 36:3043-3052.
42. Standard guide for risk-based corrective action [http://www.astm.org] *E2081-00*
43. Stärk KDC, Mortensen S, Olsen AM, Barfod K, Botner A, Lavritsen DT, Strandbygard B:Designing serological surveillance programmes to document freedom from disease with special reference to exotic viral diseases of pigs in Denmark. *Rev Sci Tech OIE* 2000, 19:715-724.
44. Suess EA, Gardner IA, Johnson WO: Hierarchical Bayesian model for prevalence inferences and determination of a country's status for an animal pathogen. *Prev Vet Med* 2002, 55:155-171.
45. Thornton R: Ambitious domesticated animal surveillance review initiated. *Biosecurity Issue* 2004, 51:6-7.
46. Thurmond MC: Conceptual foundations for infectious disease surveillance. *J Vet Diagn Invest* 2003, 15:501-514.
47. Use of risk-based decision making[http://www.epa.gov/swerust1/directiv/od961017.htm#Whatis]
48. Wagner P, Fuchs K: Sampling plan for the BHV-1 monitoring in a free region (in German). *Proceedings of the 5th International Symposium on BHV 1-, BVD- and Paratuberculosis Eradication: 9–11 March 2005; Stendal, Germany* 2005, in press.
49. Webb CR, Wilesmith JW, Simmons MM, Hoinville LJ: A stochastic model to estimate the prevalence of scrapie in Great Britain using the results of an abattoir-based survey. *Prev Vet Med* 2001, 51:269-287.
50. Ziller M, Selhorst T, Teuffert J, Kramer M, Schlüter H: Analysis of sampling strategies to substantiate freedom from disease in large areas. *Prev Vet Med* 2002, 52:333-343.

Chapter 6

Reliability of Operational Data from Pig Herds and Performance Ratings by Veterinarians and Pig Farmers Collected During Telephone Interviews for The Evaluation of a Pcv2 Piglet Vaccination

Heiko Nathues[12], Johanna Meyer-Hamme[1], Petra Maass[3], Ruediger Goessl[4], Wibke Stansen[4], Rolf Steens[5], and Elisabeth grosse Beilage[1]

[1]Field Station for Epidemiology, University of Veterinary Medicine Hannover, Foundation, Buescheler Street 9, Bakum D-49456, Germany

[2]Clinic for Swine, Department of Clinical Veterinary Medicine, Vetsuisse Faculty, University of Berne, Bremgarten Street 109a, Berne CH-3012, Switzerland

[3]Boehringer Ingelheim Animal Health GmbH, Binger Street 173, Ingelheim am Rhein D-55216, Germany

[4]Medical Data Service, Boehringer Ingelheim Pharma GmbH & Co KG, Binger Street 173, Ingelheim am Rhein D-55216, Germany[5]Boehringer Ingelheim Vetmedica GmbH, Binger Street 173, Ingelheim am Rhein D-55216, Germany

ABSTRACT

Background

The aim of the present study was to evaluate the feasibility of using a telephone survey in gaining an understanding of the possible herd and management factors influencing the performance (i.e. safety and efficacy) of a vaccine against porcine circovirus type 2 (PCV2) in a large number of herds and to estimate customers' satisfaction.

Results

Datasets from 227 pig herds that currently applied or have applied a PCV2 vaccine were analysed. Since 1-, 2- and 3-site production systems were surveyed, the herds were allocated in one of two subsets, where only applicable variables out of 180 were analysed. *Group 1* was comprised of herds with sows, suckling pigs and nursery pigs, whereas herds in *Group 2* in all cases kept fattening pigs. Overall 14 variables evaluating the subjective satisfaction with one particular PCV2 vaccine were comingled to an abstract dependent variable for further models, which was characterized by a binary outcome from a cluster analysis: good/excellent satisfaction (green cluster) and moderate satisfaction (red cluster). The other 166 variables comprised information about diagnostics, vaccination, housing, management, were considered as independent variables. In *Group 1*, herds using the vaccine due to recognised PCV2 related health problems (wasting, mortality or porcine dermatitis and nephropathy syndrome) had a 2.4-fold increased chance (1/OR) of belonging to the green cluster. In the final model for *Group 1*, the diagnosis of diseases other than PCV2, the reason for vaccine administration being other than PCV2-associated diseases and using a single injection of iron had significant influence on allocating into the green cluster ($P<0.05$). In *Group 2*, only unchanged time or delay of time of vaccination influenced the satisfaction ($P<0.05$).

Conclusion

The methodology and statistical approach used in this study were feasible to scientifically assess "satisfaction", and to determine factors influencing farmers' and vets' opinion about the safety and efficacy of a new vaccine.

BACKGROUND

Porcine circovirus type 2 (PCV2) is associated with a number of disease syndromes and in recent years, 'porcine circovirus associated diseases' (PCVD) have been considered to have severe negative impact on global pig production [1]. Before availability of PCV2 vaccines, control of PCVD was focused on assuring good management and hygiene measures as well as reducing co-infections [2]. In 2008 the first PCV2 piglet vaccine was authorized in Europe. Safety and efficacy of that vaccine was confirmed in field studies for registration according to Good Clinical Practice[3],[4]. In these negative controlled, blinded studies possible confounding factors are excluded to a large extent, allowing the detailed evaluation of vaccine safety (i.e. absence of adverse reactions, no significant negative impact on pig health, etc.) and efficacy under specific conditions. Vaccine efficacy is often determined by serological testing for specific antibodies, quantification of viral load in the serum and measuring production parameters such as daily weight gain and mortality. Due to practical reasons such controlled studies can only be performed in a limited number of herds which does not allow inclusion of the numerous factors that may have an impact on vaccine efficacy and safety in the field. The use of a telephone survey based on a subjective scaling system potentially allows the collection of data from a large number of herds representing a broad spectrum of typical conditions found in the field.

In the case of PCV2, the collection and evaluation of reliable and representative data from field trials on a larger scale is potentially complex since PCVD comprises different disease complexes[5] and can therefore have an impact on a large range of herd parameters. Since the reasons for applying a PCV2 vaccine can be varied (e.g. post weaning multi-systemic wasting syndrome, pneumonia, enteritis, etc.), the assessment of only one or two parameters may not be appropriate to sufficiently measure the vaccine efficacy. Furthermore, the collection of only a few selected herd parameters would not take into consideration the farmers' and veterinarians' subjective experiences with the vaccine, which might be a good predictor for safety and efficacy. In addition, the collection of reliable and standardised production data, as recorded in randomised and controlled clinical trials, may not be feasible when the vaccine is used in a large number of herds. In such cases 'interviews' seem to be a valuable tool to estimate safety and efficacy. When assessing individual and subjective experiences by means of interviews, investigators should take into account that the type of questioning can largely influence the validity and reliability of data[6]. Moreover, pre-tested questions for identical aspects should be used to improve the quality of information [7],[8].

The aim of the present study was to evaluate to which extent a telephone poll is in general applicable to better understand the factors influencing the performance of a vaccine in a large number of herds and to estimate customers' satisfaction (i.e. safety and efficacy of the vaccine).

METHODS

In February 2008, Ingelvac CircoFLEX® (Boehringer Ingelheim Vetmedica GmbH, Germany) received marketing authorization in the European Union. Since 2007, it was possible to use the product in Germany with a conditional license according to §17c Tierseuchengesetz (German law regulating notifiable diseases in animals and use of vaccines). The objective of this telephone survey based study was to collect and evaluate data from 2007 which could indicate 'safety' and 'efficacy', as well as to characterise factors influencing veterinarians' and farmers' satisfaction with Ingelvac CircoFLEX®.

Development and Pre-Testing of the Questionnaire

A standardised questionnaire (in German) was developed including 180 variables focussing on herd health, management, vaccination, husbandry, hygiene and on customer satisfaction (see Additional files 1 and 2). In order to receive consistently structured answers, 164 variables were assessed by closed questions (e.g. yes/no, scores from 1 = 'excellent' to 6 = 'unsatisfactory', etc.). Further experiences and occasional records were assessed by means of open questions (16 variables). For the purpose of validation, i.e. pre-testing, the principal investigator (JMH) contacted 10 farmers and their herd attending veterinarians, who had also used the PCV2 vaccine prior to authorization. They were all located in the South of Germany and their data was not included in the final analysis. During these exploratory telephone interviews, misunderstandings, unclear questions, missing variable levels, i.e. potential answers, were identified and the time needed for the individual interview, as well as the overall feasibility of the technique were evaluated. Subsequently, the questionnaire was revised according to the results of the validation process.

Inclusion and Exclusion Criteria

According to the officially granted, farm-individual permissions in six German federal states covering the area of Northern Germany (Brandenburg, Mecklenburg-Vorpommern, Niedersachsen, Nordrhein-Westfalen, Sachsen-Anhalt and Schleswig-Holstein), the PCV2 vaccine had been used in 305 herds before the product was finally authorized. The contact details of these herds (n =305) and their attending veterinarians (n =133) were provided by the manufacturer of the vaccine in compliance with German data protection rules.

All these herds including their veterinarians were proposed to be included in the study and had been contacted by the principle investigator. If farmers or veterinarians refused voluntary participation, had not used the product although they had requested it or were unavailable due to other reasons (e.g. death, etc.), these herds were excluded from the study.

Data collection

Practitioners were firstly contacted by post, explaining the aim and scope of the study, announcing that the interview will take place within the next seven days and indicating that the participation in the study is voluntary. Subsequently, veterinarians and the corresponding farmers were interviewed by the principal investigator. Each record was then entered into a digital form containing tick-boxes, drop-down menus and integer fields for coding and/or categorising given answers (Microsoft Office InfoPath 2003; www.microsoft.com *webcite*). Macros and 'if-then' logics were used to check plausibility of the data entered within each filled form.

Statistical Analysis

In a first step, all variables assessed during the interviews were assigned to the group of dependent or to the group of independent variables. Overall 14 variables evaluating the subjective satisfaction with the vaccine were assigned to the group of Y-variables (dependent variables, Table 1). The variables IL_32 and IL_3132 are assessing the (perceived) current mortality among fattening pigs in the farm and the (perceived) reduction of mortality after introduction of the vaccination in the particular farm. These questions have been answered with absolute values instead of rating on a scale from 1 to 6 and, thus are answers are not shown in Table 1. The other 166 variables comprised by various information about diagnostics, vaccination, housing, management, were considered as X-variables (Table 2).

Table 1: Y-Variables screened for feasibility of depicting the 'outcome'

Code	'Subjective' ratings* made by farmers and veterinarians (basis of the final independent variable)	Mean	SD
Questions asked to the veterinarians			

I_14	How would you estimate the overall health status of the pig herd prior to the use of the PCV2 vaccine?	3.71	1.01
I_15.1	How would you estimate the overall health status of the pig herd after starting to use the PCV2 vaccine (i.e. today!)?	2.08	0.64
I_17.1	How would you rate the handling of the vaccine?	1.96	0.40
I_18	How is the following sentence matching your opinion: "My positive expectations of the vaccine's effect in the pig herd were fulfilled"	1.95	0.65
Questions asked to the farmers			
II_22	How would you estimate the compatibility of the PCV2 vaccine?	1.88	0.62
II_23	How would you estimate the overall health status of the pig herd prior to the use of the PCV2 vaccine?	3.83	1.08
II_24.1	How would you estimate the overall health status of the pig herd after starting to use the PCV2 vaccine (i.e. today!)?	2.16	0.68
II_27	How would you estimate the uniformity of growth in the nursery unit prior to the use of the PCV2 vaccine?	3.14	0.86
II_28	How would you estimate the uniformity of growth in the nursery unit after starting to use the PCV2 vaccine?	2.22	0.47
II_29	How would you estimate the uniformity of growth in the fattening unit prior to the use of the PCV2 vaccine?	3.74	0.65
II_30	How would you estimate the uniformity of growth in the fattening unit after starting to use the PCV2 vaccine?	2.23	0.52
II_33.1	How would you rate the handling of the vaccine?	2.05	0.39
II_34.1	How would you estimate the efficacy of the vaccine?	1.97	0.73
II_35	How is the following sentence matching your opinion: 'My positive expectations of the vaccine's effect in the pig herd were fulfilled'	2.01	0.90
Calculated variables based on answers provided by veterinarians and farmers			

D_1415	[I_15.1]-[I_14] 'Change in the overall health status due to the use of a PCV2 vaccine' (veterinarians' suggestion)	1.63	0.95
D_2324	[II_24]-[II_23] 'Change in the overall health status due to the use of a PCV2 vaccine' (farmers' suggestion)	1.65	1.06
D_2728	[II_28]-[II_27] 'Change in the uniformity of growth in the nursery unit due to the use of a PCV2 vaccine' (farmers' suggestion)	0.92	0.92
D_2930	[II_30]-[II_29] 'Change in the uniformity of growth in the fattening unit due to the use of a PCV2 vaccine' (farmers' suggestion)	1.51	0.83
D_3132	'Change in the estimated mortality rate among fattening pigs due to the use of a PCV2 vaccine (farmers' suggestion)	NA	NA

*All ratings were made on a scale ranging from '1' = 'excellent' to '6' = 'unsatisfactory'/ NA = not applicable.

Nathues *et al.*

Nathues *et al. BMC Veterinary Research* 2014 10:260, doi:10.1186/s12917-014-0260-1

Table 2: Variables, which levels were assessed during telephone interviews with farmers and their veterinarians

Variable	Variable
General herd characteristics	Diagnosis of PCVD
Production type	Clinical observations
Herd size	Post mortem inspections
Production rhythm	Laboratory examinations
Purchase of animals	Time between diagnosis and first vaccination
Hygiene measures	
	Use of PCV2 vaccine
Production data	Use of PCV2 vaccines in sows
Morbidity	Use of PCV2 vaccines in piglets
Mortality	Age of piglets when vaccinated
Growth rates	Switch in timing of vaccination

	Interruption of vaccination against PCV2
Sow & gilt management*	Use of antibiotics prior and after vaccination
Acclimatisation	Time between vaccination and other measures
Vaccination	
	Experience with PCV2 vaccination
Grower & finisher management*	Compatibility
Age when moving	Perceived efficacy
Vaccination	Influence of vaccination on pig health
Other treatments	Impact of vaccination on morbidity*
	Impact of vaccination on mortality*
Intention of continuous use of the PCV2 vaccine*	Impact of vaccination on growth rate*
	Overall satisfaction with the PCV2 vaccine

*Questions were asked to farmers only.

Nathues *et al.*

Nathues *et al.* *BMC Veterinary Research* 2014 10:260, doi:10.1186/s12917-014-0260-1

In this study 1-, 2- and 3-site production systems were surveyed. For the purpose of sound analysis, the herds were further investigated in two different subsets, in which only applicable variables were further tested. *Group 1* was comprised by 171 herds, which all housed nursery pigs (farrow-to-finish herds, piglet producing herds, wean-to-finish herds and specialised nursing herds). All 163 herds in *Group 2* kept fattening pigs (mandatory) and only optional other age and production groups (farrow-to-finish herds, wean-to-finish herds, fattening herds). Overall 107 herds were analysed in both subsets, because the kept nursery pigs (*Group 1*) and fattening pigs (*Group 2*). This concept of potentially using herds in both subsets is justified by the pigs' age-dependent separation of factors that have been further analysed in each *Group*. Any potential bias due to this procedure will be discussed accordingly.

Due to the unexpected almost unanimous positive response, the statistical data analysis was done in a stepwise procedure:

- Descriptive univariate analysis for X and Y variables of the raw dataset. This dataset included all variables of the questionnaire and all answers given by farmers of 227 appropriate herds and their veterinarians.
- Descriptive univariate analysis for X and Y variables of the final dataset. In this dataset, herds with missing values in either variable were omitted because this resulted in conflicts with the tests used for further analysis (e.g. Chi-Square, regression analysis, etc.). The final analysis included 106 herds for *Group 1* and 99 herds for *Group 2*.

The subsequent analysis for the final dataset consists of the following steps:

A principal components analysis (PCA) for the responses Y to analyse the dependencies among them. The examination was carried out separately for *Group 1* and *Group 2*. Principal components explaining similarity within this data were calculated and subsequently visualised using PROC%BIPLOT macro [9].

A cluster analysis to construct distinct clusters of items showing similar scoring pattern for all responses. This approach was chosen, because a correlation analysis and modelling of X variables and individual responses or subsets is considered to yield no satisfactory results due to the low percentages of individual scores ≥4. Cluster analyses were performed for *Group 1* and *Group 2*, respectively. Herds were clustered according to the scoring given for each dependent variable (PROC FASTCLUS). Two sets of herds were guessed representing 'high satisfaction' (GREEN cluster) and 'moderate satisfaction' (RED cluster) among farmers and veterinarians. The outcome of this analysis was plotted in two dimensions obtained from the principal component analysis. Dependent variables were dropped from further data processing, when they were not adding discriminative power to the cluster analysis (i.e. they were equally expressed in both clusters).

The resulting clusters formed with variables that had not been dropped (see above) were investigated for associations between the cluster variables and X-variables in order to identify which factors might influence customer satisfaction. These bivariate relations were analysed with Fisher's exact test and the calculation of odds ratios (for 2 × 2 tables only) including confidence intervals (PROC FREQ), i.e. the comparison between GREEN and RED clusters. This procedure was run for corresponding variables of *Group 1* and *Group 2*. Variables were selected for further in-depth analysis, if the p-value of the Fisher-Exact test was <0.2, the minimum cell count in every cell was >5 and/or the association with the outcome variable was 'biologically sound'. Moreover, independent variables were dropped when missing values were observed.

A forward stepwise logistic regression model was fit to the relevant X variables considering main effects as well as two-way interactions. For the resulting final model the odds ratios of the included effects were estimated. The aim of the final analysis was to estimate the influence of the independent variables on the outcome considering potential two-way interactions among variables. Therefore, an automated stepwise logistic regression model was developed (PROC LOGISTIC, FORWARD (SLENTRY = 0.1), Option ODDSRATIO). The model was applied to data from *Group 1* and*Group 2*.

Data analysis was performed using the Statistical Analysis System (SAS®) for Windows version 8.2 and 9.2 (SAS® Institute Inc. Cary NC, USA).

This study was conducted in accordance with the research ethics requirements of the University of Veterinary Medicine Hannover. Due to the nature of the study and the low risk posed to participants, formal approval from the Ethics Committee was not a requirement at the time of the study. Potential participants were contacted by post with information explaining the purpose and nature of the study and inviting participation.

Participants were informed that their data would be kept anonymous and securely, and that any material potentially leading to identification would be removed. Subsequently, potential participants were contacted by telephone in order to provide further information. Participants were asked to provide verbal consent prior to the interview and it was made clear that by agreeing to be interviewed, they were agreeing to be part of the study.

RESULTS

Data from 243 herds were collected in this study, corresponding to a response rate of 79.7%. Reasons for non-response to this survey (n =62) were: (I) retirement, bankruptcy or death of the farmer or the veterinarian between the start of vaccination and the suggested time of the interview, (II) vaccine not used, although farmer and veterinarian had asked for a permission, (III) the herd attending veterinarian changed during the course of the evaluated time period, or (IV) the vaccine was not used for a sufficient time period (i.e. single use of the vaccine in only one batch of pigs).

Sixteen herds had to be excluded from the dataset, because either herds were selling all suckling pigs (n =4), were vaccinating only gilts during their acclimatisation period (n =4), their owner was not willing to participate in the telephone survey (n =5), or the farmer was not using the vaccine in question (n =3). In conclusion, in-depth analysis was performed based on data from 227 herds.*Group 1* was comprised of 171 herds (107 farrow-to-finish herds and 61 piglet producing herds and of 3 specialised nursery herds, all of them housing varied numbers of nursery pigs, whereas *Group 2* contained data of 163 herds, all raising grow-finish pigs (107 farrow-to-finish herds, 15 wean-to-finish herds and 41 fattening herds).

The level of 'satisfaction' with the PCV2 vaccine was consistently high in *Group 1* and *Group 2*. Particularly the efficiency, compatibility and handling of the vaccine received good to excellent evaluations by the majority of veterinarians and farmers, respectively. Due to this one-sided positive response sensitive multivariate tests (principal components analysis and cluster analysis) were used for further statistical analysis.

descriptive univariate analysis

Pre-selected independent X-variables and their levels are described in Table 3. For variables that assessed perceptions and remarks (16 open questions) a grouping of answers was not possible. Thus these 16 variables were omitted from the dataset. A further screening was conducted to identify variables associated with the 'outcome'.

Principal Component Analysis

Table 3: Independent X-variables assessed via telephone interview with veterinarians and farmers using a PCV2 vaccine in piglets prior to official release to the market

Variable	Level	Herds/level	
		(%)	(n)
General herd characteristics			
Production type	Farrow to finish	47.1	107
	Farrow to nursery	26.9	61
	Only nursery	1.3	3
	Nursery and fattening	6.6	15
	Only fattening	18.1	41
Herd size/Sowsa	≤500	78.0	131
	>500	20.8	35
	n.a.	1.2	2
Herd size/Fattening pigs b	≤500	14.7	24
	501 - 2,000	60.7	99
	>2,000	21.5	35
	n.a.	3.1	5
Sow managementa			
Acclimatisation of giltsa	Yes	61.7	103
	No	11.4	19
	Own re-breeding	21.0	35
	n.a.	6.0	10
Farrowing rhythma	1-week	42.9	72
	2-week	20.8	35
	3-week	20.8	35
	Other	15.5	26
Storage of production dataa	Electronic	89.3	150
	Hand written	10.1	17
	Nothing	0.6	1
AIAO in the farrowing unitsa	Yes	91.1	153
	No	8.9	15

Vaccination of sows [S] and gilts [G] againsta	PRRSV [S]	77.8	130
	PRRSV [G]	79.6	133
	PCV2 [S]	13.2	22
	PCV2 [G]	26.4	44
	Swine influenza virus	33.5	56
	Porcine Parvovirus & E. rhusiopathiae	98.2	164
	P. multocida	4.8	8
	E. coli	24.0	40
	Autogenous vaccines	21.0	35
Piglet management			
Age of piglets at weaning (days)a	21	44.1	74
	22 – 42	54.8	92
	n.a.	1.2	2
Age of piglets when castrateda	≤7	95.8	161
	8 – 14	4.2	7
Frequency of injecting irona	Once	67.9	114
	Twice	32.1	54
Vaccination of piglets againstc	M. hyopneumoniae	71.9	133
	using a 1-shot vaccine	40.5	75
	using a 2-shot vaccine	19.5	36
	n.a.	18.4	34
	PRRSV	31.4	58
	A. pleuropneumoniae	1.6	3
	L. intracellularis	10.3	19
	Autogenous vaccines	1.6	3
Management of fattening pigs			
AIAO in the fattening unitsb	Yes (by barn)	8.6	14
	Yes (by compartment)	77.9	127
	No	13.5	22
Storage of production datab	Electronic	16.6	27
	Hand written	81.0	132
	No	2.5	4

Disposition of low performing pigs before restockingb	Moving to younger pigs	9.8	16
	Euthanasia	9.2	15
	Hospital compartment	25.8	42
	Hospital pen	33.1	54
	Original pen	9.8	16
	Others	12.3	20
PCV2 vaccination issues			
Indication to use the vaccine (farmers' answer)	Stunted growth	59.9	136
	Respiratory diseases	26.0	59
	Enteritis	4.9	11
	PDNS	44.5	101
	Increased mortality	56.8	129
	Marketing	29.1	66
	Other reasons	33.5	72
Indication to use the vaccine (veterinarians' answer	Stunted growth	59.5	135
	Respiratory diseases	37.0	84
	Enteritis	15.4	35
	PDNS	45.8	104
	Increased mortality	47.6	108
	Marketing	26.9	61
	Other reasons	26.0	59
Duration of symptoms according to the indication before the vaccine was used for the first time (month)	<3	12.3	28
	3 – 6	4.4	10
	>6	75.3	171
	n.a.	7.9	18
Diagnostics (other than clinical examination) before vaccination	Yes	79.7	181
	No	20.3	46

Type of diagnostics	Antibody detection by ELISA	16.3	37
	of these IgM - IgG ELISA	1.3	3
	PCR	56.8	129
	Necropsy (only gross lesions)	39.2	89
	Histology	0.0	0
	Immuno-histology	1.3	3
Pathogens other than PCV2 found during these examination	Respiratory pathogens excl. PRRSV	18.1	41
	PRRSV or PRRSV & others	13.7	31
	Sc. suis or Sc. suis & others	10.6	24
	L. intracellularis & others	9.7	22
	Enteric pathogens excl. L. intracellularis	4.0	9
	Others	0.4	1
	None	43.6	99
Herd health ranking prior to the use of the PCV2 vaccine (farmers' answer)	1 (excellent)	0.0	0
	2	11.5	26
	3	22.5	51
	4	33.5	76
	5	19.4	44
	6 (unsatisfactory)	5.3	12
	k. A.	7.9	18
Herd health ranking prior to the use of the PCV2 vaccine (veterinarians' answer)	1 (excellent)	0.0	0
	2	11.5	26
	3	25.1	57
	4	35.2	80
	5	15.9	36
	6 (unsatisfactory)	3.1	7
	k. A.	9.3	21

Time between first use of the PCV2 vaccine and the telephone interview (month)	1 – 6	13.2	30
	7 – 12	73.6	167
	13 – 18	11.0	25
	n.a.	2.2	5
Age of piglets when vaccinated against PCV2 (days)	≤14	28.6	65
	15 – 21	29.1	66
	22 – 28	11.5	26
	29 – 69	8.8	20
	≥ 70	11.9	27
	Unknown*	10.1	23
Stage of production, when pigs are vaccinated against PCV2	Suckling period	63.4	144
	Nursery period	13.7	31
	Fattening period	12.8	29
	Suckling or nursery period*	10.1	23
Timing of vaccination			
Time between PCV2_ vaccination and 1st (or 2nd) vaccination against M. hyopneumoniae (days) c(farmers´ answer)	0 (in parallel)	8.7	16
	1 – 7	7.0	13
	8 – 14	4.4	10
	≥15	2.7	5
Time between PCV2_ vaccination and 1st (or 2nd) vaccination against M. hyopneumoniae (days) c(veterinarians' answer)	0 (in parallel)	22.2	41
	1 – 7	10.8	20
	8 – 14	22.7	42
	≥15	13.2	30
Time between PCV2_ vaccination and PRRSV vaccination (days) c (farmers' answer)	0 (in parallel)	8.7	16
	1 – 7	0.5	1
	8 – 14	1.1	2
	≥15	1.1	2
Time between PCV2_ vaccination and PRRSV vaccination (days)c (veterinarians' answer)	0 (in parallel)	18.9	35
	1 – 7	6.5	12
	8 – 14	3.2	6
	≥15	2.7	5

Substances applied in parallel with the PCV2 vaccine on the other side of the neck	Nothing	53.3	121
	M. hyopneumoniae vaccine	24.7	56
	PRRSV vaccine	13.2	30
	M. hyopneumoniae & PRRSV vaccine	2.2	5
	Others**	6.6	15
Castration and PCV2 vaccination in parallel	No	99.6	226
	Yes	0.4	1
Interruption of the PCV2 vaccination	No	92.5	210
	Yes	7.5	17
Actual use of the PCV2 vaccine at the time of the interview	No	10.1	23
	Yes	89.9	204
Change in the timing of PCV2 vaccination since started	No	79.7	181
	Yes	14.1	32
	n.a.	0.9	2
Use of other PCV2 vaccines than Ingelvac CircoFLEX® in piglets	No	87.7	199
	Porcilis® PCV (MSD)	6.6	15
	Suvaxyn® PCV 2 (Pfizer)	4.9	11
	Circovac® (Merial)	0.9	2
Reasons for the use of other PCV2 vaccines in piglets	Out of stock	10.1	23
	Insufficient efficacy	0.4	1
	n.a.	1.8	4

[a]only herds housing sows (n =167).

[b]only herds housing fattening pigs (n =163).

[c]only herds housing suckling and nursery pigs (n =185).

n.a.: not answered.

*pigs were either vaccinated during their suckling period or nursery period; the exact point in time was unknown.

**injection of iron, antimicrobials or other vaccines.

Nathues *et al.*

Nathues *et al.* *BMC Veterinary Research* 2014 10:260, doi:10.1186/s12917-014-0260-1

In order to analyse the relations among the responses, a principal components analysis was done for the Y variables

Group 1:

I_15.1, D_1415, I_18, II_24.1, D_2324, II_28, D_2728 , II_34.1, II_35

Group 2:

I_15.1, D_1415, I_18, II_24.1, D_2324, II_30, D_2930, II_32, D_3132, II_34.1, II_35

The results are visualized in biplots for the first two dimensions, explaining approximately 47% of the data variability for *Group 1* (Figure 1) and approximately 42% for *Group 2* (Figure 2). The plots show the correlation structure of the responses, in which several groups of two or more correlated responses can be identified.

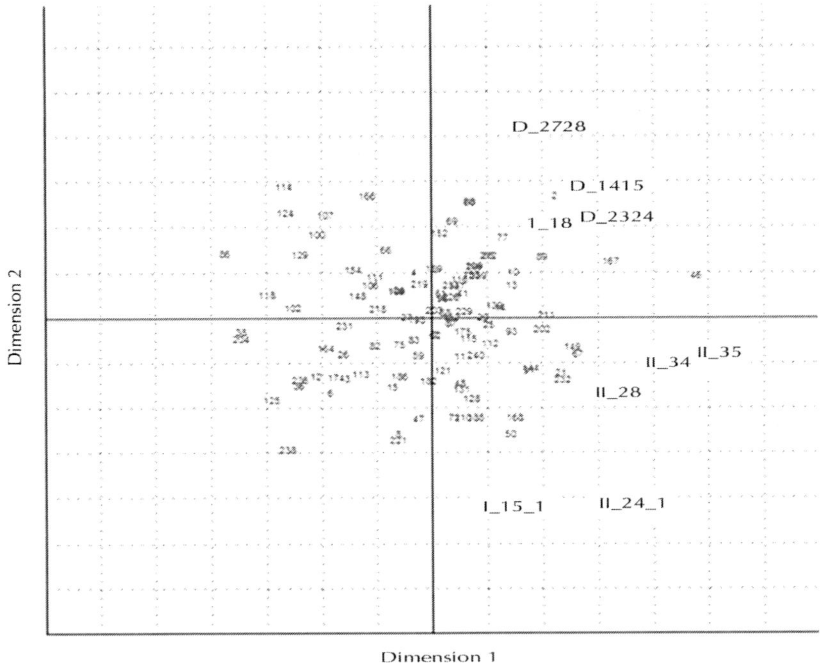

Figure 1: Bi-plot showing the results of the principal component analysis of*Group 1*. Black figures represent the dependent variables and blue figures the herds.

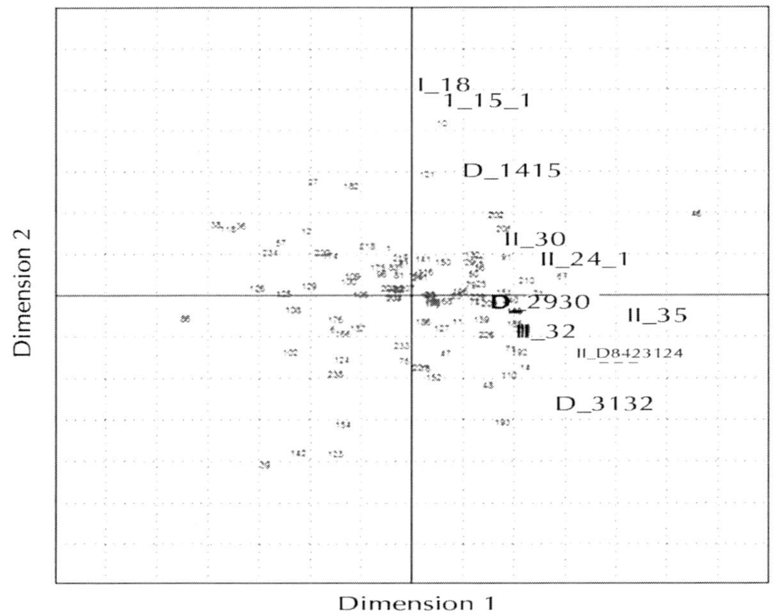

Figure 2: Bi-plot showing the results of the principal component analysis of*Group 2*. Black figures represent the dependent variables and blue figures the herds.

Some correlation between the dependent variables was observed, e.g. between II_34.1 (*'How would you estimate the efficacy of the vaccine?'*) and II_35 (*'How is the following sentence matching your opinion: 'My positive expectations of the vaccine's effect in the pig herd were fulfilled.'*), but this could be confirmed only for *Group 1* and not for *Group 2*. In contrast, the variables D_2930 (*'Change in the uniformity of growth in the fattening unit due to the use of a PCV2 vaccine'* (farmers' suggestion)') and I_15.1 (*'How would you estimate the overall health status of the pig herd after starting to use the PCV2 vaccine (i.e. today!)?'*) do not seem to be correlated. Conclusively, the results of the principal component analysis did not lead to a further reduction of dependent variables or selection of a representative dependent variable, because of the correlation structure amongst them.

Cluster Analysis

The clustering procedure was done for the same response as for the principal component analysis via the SAS® procedure PROC FASTCLUS

(SAS/STAT® (1999) - *User's Guide Version 8*, SAS® Institute Inc – Cary NC) using the k-means method. The applied procedure resulted in two distinct clusters for each group:

GREEN cluster with n =60 for *Group 1* and n =64 for *Group 2*,

RED cluster with n =46 for *Group 1* and n =35 for *Group 2*.

As a graphical representation of the clustering results, the GREEN and RED cluster were coloured in the PCA biplots (Figures 3 and 4) showing a quite good cluster separation in the first two dimensions (for detailed results see Additional files 1 and 2). With exception of I_15.1 (*'How would you estimate the overall health status of the pig herd after starting to use the PCV2 vaccine (i.e. today!)?'*), on average the GREEN cluster has lower (='better') scores than the RED cluster and the highest differences can be seen for the responses II_34.1 (*'How would you estimate the efficacy of the vaccine?'*) and II_35 (*'How is the following sentence matching your opinion: 'My positive expectations of the vaccine's effect in the pig herd were fulfilled'*).

Selection of Independent Variables and Test of Association

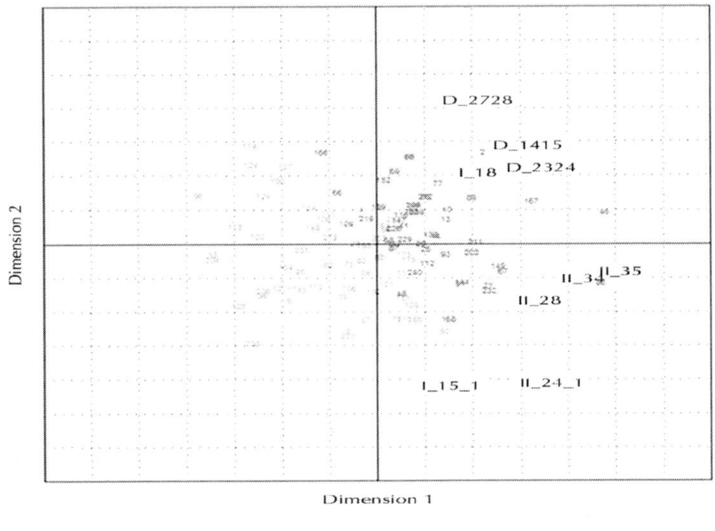

Figure 3: Bi-plot showing the results of a principal component analysis including response clustering for*Group 1*. Black figures represent the dependent variables and green/red figures the herds.

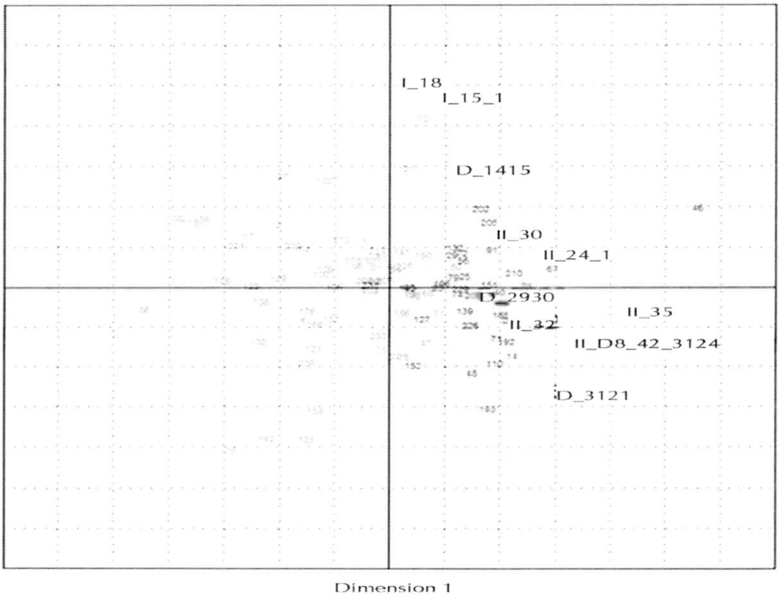

Figure 4: Bi-plot showing the results of a principal component analysis including response clustering for*Group 2*. Black figures represent the dependent variables and green/red figures the herds.

Table 4 summarizes the p-values of the individual Fisher's tests comparing GREEN versus RED cluster for the corresponding X-variables. Overall eight X-Variables with p-value <0.2 were selected for further modelling analysis.

Logistic Regression Model

Table 4: p-values of the individual Fisher tests comparing green versus red cluster

Independent X-variable	p-value (Fisher test)	
	Group 1	Group 2

Reasons for using the vaccine were either wasting, mortality or PDNS, but were not respiratory diseases, enteritis and/or marketing. (veterinarians' answer)	0.423	0.144
Diagnosis of other diseases than PCVD	0.071	1.000
Acclimatisation of gilts	0.258	na
Vaccination of sows against PRRSV	0.395	na
Vaccination of gilts against PRRSV	0.334	na
Frequency of iron injection in piglets	0.040	na
Age of piglets when vaccinated against PCV2	0.075	na
Reasons for using the vaccine were either wasting, mortality or PDNS, but were not respiratory diseases, enteritis and/or marketing (farmers' answer)	0.031	0.531
Overall health status of the pig herd prior to the use of the PCV2 vaccine (veterinarians' answer)	0.001	0.123
Overall health status of the pig herd prior to the use of the PCV2 vaccine (farmers' answer)	0.000	0.000
Time between first use of the PCV2 vaccine and the telephone interview	na	0.725
Change in the timing of PCV2 vaccination since started	na	0.058
Actual use of the PCV2 vaccine at the time of the interview (veterinarians' answer)	na	0.343
Actual use of the PCV2 vaccine at the time of the interview (farmers' answer)	na	0.285

na: not applicable.

Nathues *et al.*

Nathues *et al. BMC Veterinary Research* 2014 10:260, doi:10.1186/s12917-014-0260-1

On the basis of the cluster analyses and the selected eight X-variables two logistic regression models were used for *Group 1* and *Group 2*, respectively, with the FORWARD (SLENTRY =0.1) stepwise model selection option allowing for the inclusion of main effects and two-way interaction terms. Not considered in this selection were the variables II_23 (*'How would you estimate the overall health status of the pig herd prior to the use of the PCV2 vaccine?' farmer's answer*) and I_14 (*'How would you estimate the overall health status of the pig herd prior to the use of the PCV2 vaccine?' veterinarian's answer*). The procedure led to the following X variables in a final model

Group 1: 'Diagnosis of other diseases than PCVD', 'Frequency of iron injection in piglets', 'Reasons for using the vaccine', combination of 'Diagnosis of other diseases than PCVD' and 'Reasons for using the vaccine'

Group 2: 'Actual use of the PCV2 vaccine at the time of the interview', 'Time of vaccinating piglets not changed or changed to another point in piglets' life'

Overall, only a few variables could be identified as influencing veterinarians' and farmers' 'satisfaction' with the PCV2 vaccine. These variables were not identical in *Group 1* and *Group 2*(Tables 5 and 6). This indicates that satisfaction among piglet producers, owners of only fattening pigs and farmers operating a 1-site production system may be influenced by different criteria.

Table 5: Odds ratio estimates and 95% confidence intervals for the 'GREEN cluster' in the final model for*Group 1*

Independent X-variable	OR	95% CI
Only one application of iron in suckling pigs	2.83	1.18-6.80
No findings of other diseases than PCVD, when reasons for using the vaccine were respiratory disease, enteritis and/or marketing	0.16	0.05-0.56
No findings of other diseases than PCVD, when reasons for using the vaccine were wasting, mortality and/or PDNS, but not respiratory disease, enteritis and/or marketing	1.32	0.35-5.05
Reasons for using the vaccine were neither wasting nor mortality nor PDNS, but were respiratory diseases, enteritis and/or marketing. Simultaneously, no findings of other diseases in the herd	0.10	0.02-0.45

Reasons for using the vaccine were neither wasting nor mortality nor PDNS, but were respiratory diseases, enteritis and/or marketing. Simultaneously, findings of other diseases in the herd	0.84	0.29-2.41

Numbers in bold font indicate that the odds ratios are significantly different from one at the 5-percent level of significance.

Nathues *et al.*

Nathues *et al. BMC Veterinary Research* 2014 10:260, doi:10.1186/s12917-014-0260-1

Table 6: Odds ratio estimates and 95% confidence intervals for the 'GREEN cluster' identified in the final model for*Group 2*

Independent X-variable	OR	95% CI
Time of vaccinating piglets not changed or change to a later point in piglets' life instead of earlier point in time	10.29	1.56-67.9
Time of vaccinating piglets not changed instead of changing to an earlier point in piglets' life	5.00	1.18-21.1
PCV2 vaccine still in use instead of no longer in use	5.02	0.67-37.6

Numbers in bold font indicate that the odds ratios are significantly different from one at the 5-percent level of significance.

Nathues *et al.*

Nathues *et al. BMC Veterinary Research* 2014 10:260, doi:10.1186/s12917-014-0260-1

Tables 5 and 6 show the p-values and odds ratio estimates for the final models including 95% confidence intervals. The odds ratio estimates had been calculated with the ODDSRATIO option of the SAS® procedure PROC LOGISTIC available only in Version 9.2.

DISCUSSION

The primary aim of the present study was to evaluate the reliability of operational data from pig herds and performance ratings by veterinarians and farmers collected during telephone interviews for the assessment of the 'safety' and 'efficacy' of a specific PCV2 vaccination in piglets. To the best knowledge of the authors, the feasibility of a telephone survey as an instrument for examining different drivers of using a vaccine in livestock, and as for examining its safety and efficacy in a large number of herds has not been described before.

Telephone interviews with customers, usually aimed to gather information about satisfaction with products or to explore the expectations of clients, are a frequently applied technique in the context of market research [10]. In contrast, veterinary research, especially in livestock animals, is mainly linked with classical on-farm interviews followed by an examination of the animals, the environment and the management. This procedure is currently ranked as the 'gold standard' and scientific reports based exclusively on interviews by telephone are rarely published. Interestingly, data obtained during a face to face interview can be of lower quality than such data collected via a telephone interview, because in the anonymous situation of a telephone call, the interviewees are more likely to give answers reflecting the reality [8]. Moreover, the latter technique is more cost effective than on-site visits and, if a considerable number of cases is investigated, is more time efficient [6]. The present study was to be performed under economic constraints as well as during a short time period. Therefore, a telephone survey was considered as the method of choice.

The response rate of about 80%, achieved in the present study, was considered to be highly satisfactory. Analysing the reasons for non-responding, it can be assumed that no bias was introduced by those veterinarians and farmers who had refused their participation. Other studies applying telephone interviews as the investigational tool have reported significantly lower response rates, but were still seen as relevant [8],[11].

Measures of the safety and efficacy of the PCV2 vaccine involved were extrapolated from parameters assessing farmers' and veterinarians' overall 'satisfaction' with the product. This approach was chosen, because the comparison of this subjective data is more reliable than using production data (e.g. weight gain, feed consumption, etc.), if these data have not been determined under standardized conditions [12]. Marking with a nominal scale from 1 (excellent) to 6 (unsatisfactory) usually represents accurately the personal experience with a product.

Calculating the increase or decrease after the introduction of any procedure allows for a comparison of relative values describing the effect of this procedure on the corresponding parameter. It is noteworthy that the relative values can be biased by professional marketing activities as has been shown for pharmaceuticals in human medicine [13], but this would usually affect only the magnitude and not the trend of the figures.

In order to determine the 'satisfaction' ('dependent variable') and to explore related parameters ('independent variables'), two different statistical methods were tested for their suitability to separate different multivariate outcomes. The principal components analysis did not lead to a further reduction of the dependent variables or the identification of representative dependent variables. The cluster analysis resulted in a sufficient separation of highly and less satisfied cases. Further tests for association and modelling approaches were conducted using the two clusters, which had been identified with this descriptive method. In this specific study the principal component analysis was not able to reduce the dependent variables or identify representative dependent variables due to the almost unanimous positive response when asked for the satisfaction with the PCV2 vaccination. However, for a similar type of study, the same set of statistical methods would be applied in the same order and a principal component analysis might in this case result in a reduction of the dependent variables, which would be used as input for a subsequent cluster analysis and/or modelling approach.

Interestingly, only very few of the parameters listed in Tables 2 and 3 were associated with the overall satisfaction with the vaccine. Finally, three parameters for *Group 1* and two for *Group 2*were identified as 'risk factors' influencing the overall 'satisfaction' with the vaccine (Table 5 and6). Farmers and veterinarians were less satisfied, when reasons for using the vaccine were not PCVD, wasting and/or mortality, but any other disease in the farm, which had not been properly diagnosed. These findings are conclusive since any effect of the vaccine in the absence of PCVD, or other diseases associated with PCV2 infection [14], is unlikely. Hence, these biologically sound results underline the suitability of the methods used in this study. The apparently protective effect of applying iron to piglets only once instead of twice cannot be explained. In humans, iron overload is associated with reduced phagocytosis by macrophages and monocytes [15] and a decrease of the efficiency of the unspecific immune system [16]. Whether these effects also occur in pigs and could impact the efficacy of any vaccination remains speculative. In *Group 2* the 'satisfaction' with the vaccine was associated with the time when the pigs were vaccinated. Taking the large confidence intervals into account, the results should be interpreted with caution, if at all[17].

Overall there was very little influence on the generally excellent satisfaction rate found in this study, which is in line with the PCV2 vaccine evaluated in this study having the highest global market shares as shown by market research figures [18]. The overall approach used in this study was feasible to scientifically assess 'satisfaction', and to determine factors influencing farmers' and veterinarians' opinion about 'safety', 'efficacy' and handling of a new vaccine. Since no strong associations were found between 'dissatisfaction of users' and the various parameters assessed in this study, it can be assumed that vaccine's safety profile is high and that potential factors leading to a decreased efficacy of the product do not play any role under field conditions.

CONCLUSIONS

It was demonstrated that a telephone survey using standardised questionnaires may be an efficient method to investigate safety and efficacy aspects of vaccines as well as customer satisfaction on a broad basis. However, due to the unexpected almost unanimous positive response to the vaccine, the present study does not allow a conclusive evaluation of the use of telephone surveys in general. Nonetheless, this study describes a suitable example of how data from field trials including a large number of herds could be assessed and analysed.

AUTHORS' CONTRIBUTIONS

HN, JMH and EGB designed the study and drafted the roadmap. JMH conducted the interviews and digitalised the data. HN, JMH, PM and RS structured and analysed the data. RG and WS supported the statistical analysis. HN, JMH, PM, RS and EGB critically reviewed the results and discussed their implication for the hypothesis of this study. HN drafted the manuscript. JMH, RG, WS, PM, RS and EGB approved the manuscript. All authors read and approved the final manuscript.

ACKNOWLEDGMENTS

We thank the farmers and the veterinarians, who contributed to this study, for their valuable time. This study was financially supported by Boehringer Ingelheim Vetmedica.

REFERENCES

1. Segales J, Allan GM, Domingo M: Porcine circovirus diseases. *Anim Health Res Rev* 2005, 6:119-142.
2. Madec F, Eveno E, Morvan P, Hamon L, Blanchard P, Cariolet R, Amenna N, Morvan H, Truong C, Mahe D, Albina E, Jesting A: Post-weaning multisystemic wasting syndrome (PMWS) in pigs in France: clinical observations from follow-up studies on affected farms. *Livestock Prod Sci* 2000, 63:223-233.
3. Fachinger V, Bischoff R, Jedidia B, Saalmueller A, Elbers K: The effect of vaccination against porcine circovirus type 2 in pigs suffering from porcine respiratory disease complex. *Vaccine* 2008, 26:1488-1499.
4. Kixmoller M, Ritzmann M, Eddicks M, Saalmueller A, Elbers K, Fachinger V: Reduction of PMWS-associated clinical signs and co-infections by vaccination against PCV2. *Vaccine* 2008, 26:3443-3451
5. Segales J: Porcine circovirus type 2 (PCV2) infections: clinical signs, pathology and laboratory diagnosis. *Virus Res* 2012, 164(1–2):10-19.
6. Seipel C, Rieker P: *Integrative Sozialforschung: Konzepte und Methoden der qualitativen und quantitativen empirischen Forschung*. Weinheim und Muenchen, Juventa Verlag, Germany; 2003.
7. Cameron A, Sergeant E, Baldock C: The AusVet series in epidemiological skills for Animals Health Professionals. In *Data Management for Animal Health*. AusVet Animal Health Services, Brisbane, Australia; 2004.
8. Stege H, Christensen J, Nielsen JP, Willeberg P: Data-quality issues and alternative variable-screening methods in a

questionnairebased study on subclinical Salmonella enterica infection in Danish pig herds. *Prev Vet Med* 2001, 48:35-54.

9. Friendly M: *System for Statistical Graphics*. Carey, NC, USA, SAS Insitute; 1991.
10. Kuss A: *Marketing-Einführung*. Betriebswirtschaftlicher Verlag Gabler Fachverlage GmbH, Wiesbaden, Germany; 2006.
11. Atteslander P: *Methoden der empirischen Sozialforschung*. Verlag deGruyter, Berlin, Germany; 2003.
12. Dohoo IR, Ducrot C, Fourichon C, Donald A, Hurnik D: An overview of techniques for dealing with large numbers of independent variables in epidemiologic studies. *Prev Vet Med* 1997, 29:221-239.
13. Grande D, Frosch DL, Perkins AW, Kahn BE: Effect of Exposure to Small Pharmaceutical Promotional Items on Treatment Preferences. *Arch Intern Med* 2009, 169:887-893.
14. Opriessnig T: Porcine circovirus type 2: Current understanding of pathogenesis and role of coinfections. In Proceedings of the 40thAnn. Meeting Am. Assoc. Swine Vet., Vol. 1, Volume 1. Dallas, USA: AASV; 2009:491–498.
15. Walker E, Walker S: Effects of iron overload in the immune system. *Ann Clin Lab Sci* 2000, 30:354-365.
16. Ward CG, Bullen JJ, Rogers HJ: Iron and Infection: New Development and Their Implications. *J Traumata* 1996, 41:356-364.
17. du Prell JP, Hommel G, Roehrig B, Blettner M: Konfidenzintervall oder p-Wert? *Deutsches Aerzteblatt* 2009, 106:335-339.
18. Hardge T, Koerk C: Global vaccine market driven by PCV2 vaccination. In *Asian Pork Market*. Boehringer Ingelheim, Tsukuba, Japan; 2009:28-29.

Chapter 7

A Four Year Longitudinal Sero-Epidemiological Study of Bovine Herpesvirus Type-1 (BHV-1) in adult Cattle in 107 Unvaccinated Herds in South West England

Kerry A Woodbine, Graham F Medley, Stephen J Moore, Ana M Ramirez-Villaescusa, Sam Mason, and Laura E Green

Department of Biological Science, University of Warwick, Coventry, CV4 7AL, UK

For all author emails, please log on

ABSTRACT

Background

Bovine herpesvirus type-1 (BHV-1) is an important pathogen of cattle that presents with a variety of clinical signs, including the upper respiratory tract infection infectious bovine rhinotracheitis (IBR). A seroepidemiological study of BHV-1 antibodies was conducted in England from 2002 – 2004: 29,782 blood samples were taken from 15,736 cattle from 114 herds which were visited on up to three occasions. Antibody concentration was measured using a commercial ELISA. Farm management information was collected using an interview questionnaire, and herd size and cattle movements were obtained from the cattle tuberculosis testing database and the British Cattle Movement Service. Hierarchical statistical models were used to investigate associations between cattle and herd variables and the continuous outcome percentage positive (PP) values from the ELISA test in unvaccinated herds.

Results

There were 7 vaccinated herds, all with at least one seropositive bovine. In unvaccinated herds 83.2% had at least one BHV-1 seropositive bovine, and the mean cattle and herd BHV-1 seroprevalence were 42.5% and 43.1% respectively. There were positive associations between PP value, age, herd size, presence of dairy cattle. Adult cattle in herds with grower cattle had lower PP values than those in herds without grower cattle. Purchased cattle had significantly lower PP values than homebred cattle, whereas cattle in herds that were totally restocked after the foot-and-mouth epidemic in 2001 had significantly higher PP values than those in continuously stocked herds. Samples taken in spring and summer had significantly lower PP values than those taken in winter, whereas those taken in autumn had significantly higher PP values than those taken in winter. The risks estimated from a logistic regression model with a binary outcome (seropositive yes/no) were similar.

Conclusion

The prevalence of BHV-1 seropositivity in cattle and herds has increased since the 1970s. Although the study population prevalence of BHV-1 was temporally stable during study period, the associations between serological status and cattle age, herd size, herd type, presence of young stock and restocked versus continuously stocked herds indicate that there is heterogeneity between herds and so potential for further spread of BHV-1 within and between herds.

BACKGROUND

Bovine herpesvirus type-1 (BHV-1) is a member of the family Herpesviridae, subfamilyAlphaherpesvirinae. It is an important pathogen of cattle worldwide [1]. Infection with BHV-1 causes a variety of clinical diseases including infectious bovine rhinotracheitis (IBR) (BHV-1 subtypes 1 and 2a), infectious pustular vulvovaginitis, infectious pustular balanoposthitis (BHV-1 subtype 2b) and encephalitis (BHV-1 subtype 3) [2]. Conventional serological assays cannot distinguish between antigenic serotypes of BHV-1.

BHV-1 generally infects cattle greater than 6 months of age once maternal immunity has waned[3]. Clinical signs associated with infection include nasal discharge, conjunctivitis, fever, inappetance, milk drop, abortion and, sometimes, death, although sub-clinical infection is possible[4,5]. The virus is shed in secretions from the eyes, nose and reproductive organs. After initial infection and disease, cattle become carriers of the virus which becomes latent in the trigeminal or sacral ganglia. Reactivation of the virus may occur when cattle are stressed [4] and virus can then be transmitted to susceptible cattle. Infection can occur indirectly through contaminated material and wind borne particles [2].

BHV-1 has been in Great Britain (GB) since the 1960s [6]. IBR was first confirmed in GB in 1961[7,8], but was not considered clinically important in GB until an outbreak of disease in Scotland in the late 1970s caused by a virulent strain of BHV-1 (subtype 1) [9-11]. In England and Wales, the overall prevalence of BHV-1 seropositive cattle was 2.1% in 1963 [6], rising to 15.1% of dairy and 16.8% of suckler cattle over 2 yrs of age in Norfolk in 1991 [12], and by 1992 BHV-1 antibodies were detected in 34% of cattle herds in the UK [13].

The reported risk factors for the presence of BHV-1 antibodies in cattle in the Netherlands included a large herd size, dairy herds with beef/veal cattle, a high density of herds in the municipality [14], purchasing cattle, cattle participating in shows, professional visitors not using farm protective clothing and herds situated close to other BHV-1 positive herds [15]. In Belgium, seropositivity was associated with increasing cattle age and herd size and purchased cattle had a higher probability of being infected than homebred cattle [16,17].

This paper presents the largest longitudinal study of BHV-1 seropositivity in cattle in the UK, and its association with cattle age, birthplace, herd type and size.

METHODS

Source of Data

The data used in this paper came from 114 dairy and/or suckler herds in south west England. Farms were visited between 2002 and 2006 and were located within the Randomised Badger Culling Trial (RBCT) [18]. In addition, the study included some farms that had been depopulated in 2001 as a result of the foot-and-mouth disease (FMD) epidemic [19] and subsequently repopulated. All the farmers agreed to participate and allow their breeding cattle to be sampled.

Samples of blood (up to 10 ml) were collected under Home Office licence from all accessible cattle over 2 years of age at three routine visits, at approximately one year intervals. A subset of herds (n = 15) had a whole herd test, i.e. blood samples were collected from cattle of all ages, prompted by the presence of an animal persistently infected (PI) with bovine viral diarrhoea virus (BVDV). Four herds had a whole herd test instead of a routine third visit; otherwise whole herd tests were additional to routine tests.

All blood samples were centrifuged at the University of Warwick at 3220 g for 15 minutes, and serum was removed and frozen at -20°C.

Farmers completed an interview questionnaire between 17th June 2003 and 18th February 2004 to obtain information on clinical signs of infectious bovine rhinotracheitis (IBR) disease and use of a BHV-1 vaccine. Four out of 114 farmers did not complete the questionnaire.

At each visit, the unique identity of cattle was recorded from their ear tag and linked to the relevant blood sample. When appropriate, freeze brand numbers were also recorded. The ear tag was matched to the individual cattle data on the British Cattle Movement Service (BCMS) to obtain/confirm the following: the date of birth, whether the animal was homebred or purchased, breed and sex. More than 99% of cattle were matched within the BCMS dataset. The main reason that cattle were not matched was because they were born before 2001, when it was not compulsory to record cattle birth dates. Herd size was estimated from the cattle tuberculosis testing data (VetNet database), and validated during farm visits.

All data were entered into a relational database (PostgreSQL, PostgreSQL Global Development Group) using Microsoft Access (Microsoft Corp. US) as a front end. All data were screened for errors. When data mismatches were detected, data were re-checked to determine the source of the mismatch and where possible this was corrected.

Serological Test and Interpretation

The presence of BHV-1 specific antibodies (IgG_1) was detected using the SVANOVIR® IBR-Ab (Svanova Biotech AB, Uppsala Sweden) indirect enzyme-linked immunosorbent assay (ELISA). All testing was completed according to the kit instructions. Internal controls were included on each plate to control for batch to batch variation. All samples were run in duplicate, and all testing was completed at the University of Warwick. Positive samples were re-tested when the duplicates were more than 0.25 optical densities (OD) units apart or when the OD of the positive controls was more than 0.2 OD units apart. The sensitivity and specificity of the serological kit to the serum neutralisation test have been reported as 97.4% and 92.4% respectively [20]. BHV-1 antibody concentration was calculated as the percentage of the positive control serum (PP) using the following calculation:

$$PPSample = \frac{OD_{Sample}}{OD_{PositiveControl}}$$

The PP values ranged from -1.01 to 2.81. A sample was defined as positive when the OD > cut-off and negative when the OD < cut-off. The cut offs were:

Cut-off = 0.2 when $OD_{Negative\ control} \times 2.5 < 0.2$

Cut-off = $OD_{Negative\ control} \times 2.5$ when $OD_{Negative\ control} \times 2.5 \geq 0.0032$

Vaccination

It was not possible to differentiate antibodies stimulated through vaccination from those from natural infection and so the 7 vaccinated herds were excluded from the analysis.

Datasets

The full serological dataset consisted of 29,782 ELISA results. Date of birth and identification of cattle were not available for 1,838 and 344 observations respectively. For the purpose of this study, two datasets (A and B) were used. Dataset A included all serological results for all cattle from herds that were not vaccinated against BHV-1 for all visits (26,918 samples, 14,243 cattle, 107 herds). Dataset B was a subset of Dataset A and included all serological results from cattle >2 years of age from the three routine visits and 4 whole herd visits (24,182 samples, 12,764 cattle, 107 herds).

Outcome variables

A herd was defined as BHV-1 seropositive when at least one cow in the herd was above the cut off for BHV-1 on at least one occasion.

Cattle were defined as BHV-1 seropositive when above the cut off for BHV-1 at least once.

The herd BHV-1 seroprevalence was calculated at each visit as the number of seropositive cattle in the herd divided by the total number of cattle tested.

Seroconversion was defined in a herd when at least one cow changed from being seronegative to seropositive between two visits.

Two outcomes were modelled to investigate associations between BHV-1 seropositivity and herd and cow variables. These were the continuous outcome PP, and a binary (positive/negative) outcome (seropositive yes/no).

The Explanatory Variables

The variables listed in Table 1 were tested as fixed effects. The variables triplet code (i.e. the form of badger control in the RBCT), herd restocking status after the 2001 FMD epidemic and farm geographical location were forced into the models because they formed part of the study design.

Table 1: The explanatory variables in the repeated measures multi-level model (Tables 3 and 4)

Explanatory variable	Variable defined
Triplet Code	Treatment in the Random Badger Culling Trial (RBCT)
Restocked	Herd was depopulated due to the foot-and-mouth (FMD) epidemic in 2001
Geographical area (farm location)	Geographical area, which the farm was situated in, categorised as Area A-(Gloucestershire, Herefordshire/Worcestershire), Area B-(northeast Devon, south Somerset), Area C-(northwest Devon, northeast Cornwall)
Cattle age (years)	In yearly intervals from 2 years old up to 10 years and over
Herd size	Taken from the VetNet database the average number of cattle present in the herd during the study period
Birthplace of replacement cattle	Cattle were homebred (tested in natal herd) or purchased (tested in herd different from natal herd)
Dairy cattle	Yes or no dairy cattle were present in the herd

Grower cattle	Yes or no grower cattle were present in the herd
Season	Time when visit took place. Winter (December, January and February), Spring (March, April and May), Summer (June, July and August) and Autumn (September, October and November)

Woodbine et al. BMC Veterinary Research 2009 5:5 doi:10.1186/1746-6148-5-5

Statistical Analysis

Associations between the outcomes and herd and animal factors were initially screened using Mann-Whitney and chi-squared tests. Variables with a significance value of <0.20 in the univariate analysis were tested in two multi-level models: one with a continuous outcome of PP value and one with a binary outcome of seropositive yes/no. There were three hierarchical levels in the models: repeated measure at each visit (level 1), clustered by cow (level 2), and herd (level 3) to control for the dependency between repeated measures within cattle and cattle within herds. The multivariable models were built using both manual forward selection and backwards elimination.

The models took the form:

$$Y_{ijk} = \beta X_0 + \beta X_k + \beta X_{jk} + \beta X_{ijk} + v_k + u_{jk} + e_{ijk} \qquad (1)$$

where Y_{ijk} is the PP value or seropositivity value at visit i from cow j in herd k. βX_0 is the intercept,βX is a series of vectors of fixed effect varying at the herd (k), cattle (jk) and visit (ijk), $v_k + u_{jk}$ are the variances at the herd and cattle levels, and e_{ijk} is the residual variance.

The model fit was assessed by plotting the raw, standardised and deletion residuals, and the leverage and influence for each random effect and all fixed effects were also assessed [21]. The detection of outliers in the models was completed using a top-down approach [22]: outliers at level 3 (herds) were examined first, and then the lower level clusters (cattle and visits). A model which included only the seropositive herds in Dataset B was also built using the procedure above.

Correlations between the explanatory variables were investigated using chi-squared tests. Variables that were significantly ($P < 0.01$) associated with each other were noted to help with interpretation. All analyses were done using MLwiN version 2.02 (Centre for Multilevel Modelling, Bristol, UK) [23].

RESULTS

Descriptive statistics

Study visits

All 107 unvaccinated herds were visited at least once, 96 were visited twice and 95 were visited on three occasions, generating 9136, 8099 and 7850 serum samples, respectively. A further 1833 blood samples were collected from additional visits or because of a whole herd test and/or cattle were under 2 years of age.

Vaccination and Clinical Signs

The median herd size of vaccinated herds was 274; in contrast, the median herd size of unvaccinated herds was 185. The median herd size of unvaccinated seronegative and seropositive herds was 58 and 193, respectively. Nine percent (10/114) of farmers reported that they had seen clinical signs of IBR in their herd in the past, and two of these farmers also reported that they now vaccinated their cattle. All vaccinated herds had at least one seropositive animal compared with 83.2% of unvaccinated herds with at least one seropositive animal. The mean within-herd seroprevalence in vaccinated herds was 74.9% compared with 43.2% in unvaccinated herds.

Herd and Cattle BHV-1 Seroprevalence

There were 89 herds (83.2%, 95% CI, 77.6% – 88.8%) with at least one BHV-1 seropositive bovine on at least one occasion (Table 2). A total of 6,993 cattle (49.0%, 95% CI, 48.2% – 49.8%) always tested negative, and 6,056 always tested positive (42.5%, 95% CI, 41.7% – 43.3%) (Table2). Nine hundred and eighty five cattle from 53 herds seroconverted between one test and the next, indicating transmission of virus within these herds. The mean and median herd BHV-1 seroprevalence were 43.2% and 40.0% (range, 0.9% – 99.2%) (Table 2). When only the herds where seroconversion had occurred were analysed, the mean and median within herd seroprevalence were 52.9% and 57.1% (range, 2.1% – 99.2%) (Table 2). There was a large statistically significant difference between the median seroprevalence in herds where cattle had seroconverted (57.1%) and those where they had not (10.6%): *U* = 1908; P <0.05, (Mann-Whitney *U*-test).

Table 2: Number and percentage of seropositive BHV-1 herds and cattle by visit type for Dataset A (26,918 samples, 14,243 cattle, 107 herds), and herd BHV-1 antibody seroprevalence for positive herds only

Visit	Positive herds		Positive cattle		Herd seroprevalence for positive herds		
	Number	%	Number	%	Median	Mean	Prevalence range
1st routine visit	85	79.4	4,228	46.3	40.0 (51.7)	42.8 (50.9)	0.9 – 95.9 (2.1 – 95.9)
2nd routine visit	74	77.1	3,918	48.4	45.9 (60.2)	43.1 (52.7)	2.7 – 95.9 (2.9 – 95.9)
3rd routine visit/3rd routine and whole herd visit	74	77.9	4,495	50.0	40.4 (59.9)	43.6 (55.1)	2.4 – 99.2 (2.4 – 99.2)
Other non-routine visits	5	38.5	342	49.2	86.6 (73.2)	77.8 (73.4)	43.8 – 100.0 (43.8 – 100.0)
Combined	89	83.0	7,250	51.0	74.0 (74.0)	74.0 (74.0)	73.1 – 75.0 (73.1 – 75.0)

The results for herds where cattle seroconverted are in brackets.

Woodbine et al. BMC Veterinary Research 2009 5:5 doi:10.1186/1746-6148-5-5

Given the reported sensitivity and specificity of the ELISA, approximately 700 and 2,046 cattle tests during the study are expected to be false negatives and false positives, respectively. There were 124 cattle that tested positive and then negative at subsequent visits. In addition, 85 cattle changed serological status twice: 25 cattle tested positive, negative than positive and 60 cattle tested negative, positive than negative. Note that we assume that antibody positivity remains for life after infection; if antibody titre wanes with time since infection, then a conversion from positive to negative might reflect a true status rather than a test failure.

Univariate Associations with BHV-1 Antibody Seroprevalence

The seroprevalence of antibodies against BHV-1 increased with age (Figure 1). The seroprevalence was consistently higher in adult cattle in herds where there was seroconversion but the same trend with age was present in seropositive herds where no cattle seroconverted (Figure 1). The decline in antibody from 6 months of age and seroconversion at approximately 13 months of age is indicative of loss of maternal immunity followed by active seroconversion (Figure 1). The seroprevalence of antibodies was higher in large herds where cattle seroconverted compared with large herds where no cattle seroconverted. There was also a trend that seroprevalence was higher as herd size increased in herds where cattle seroconverted; this was not apparent where there was no seroconversion (Figure 2). There was a statistically significant difference between the medians of the two groups in Figure 2 ($U = 0$; $P < 0.05$, Mann-Whitney U-test).

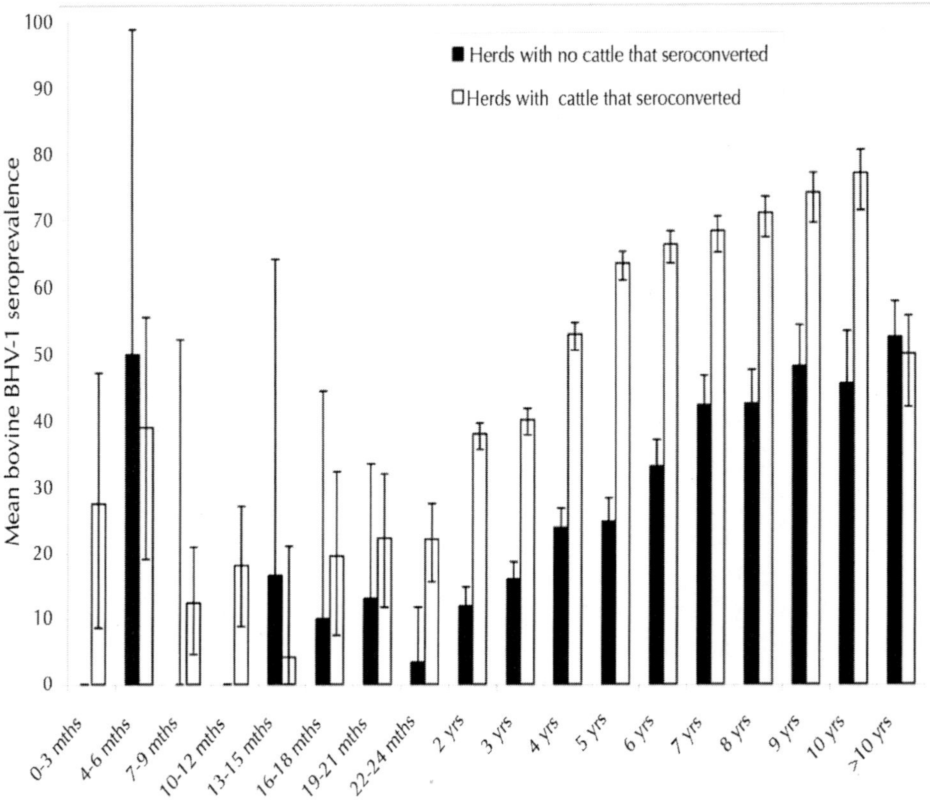

Figure 1: Unadjusted age-specific profile of the mean BHV-1 antibody seroprevalence and 95% CI by quarter year (up to 2 years old) and year (after 2 years old) for seropositive herds. Herds are dichotomised by presence of seroconversion in the period of study. All cattle greater than 10 years of age were categorised in one age group. Data came from all visits to BHV-1 unvaccinated herds (Dataset A, see methods section).

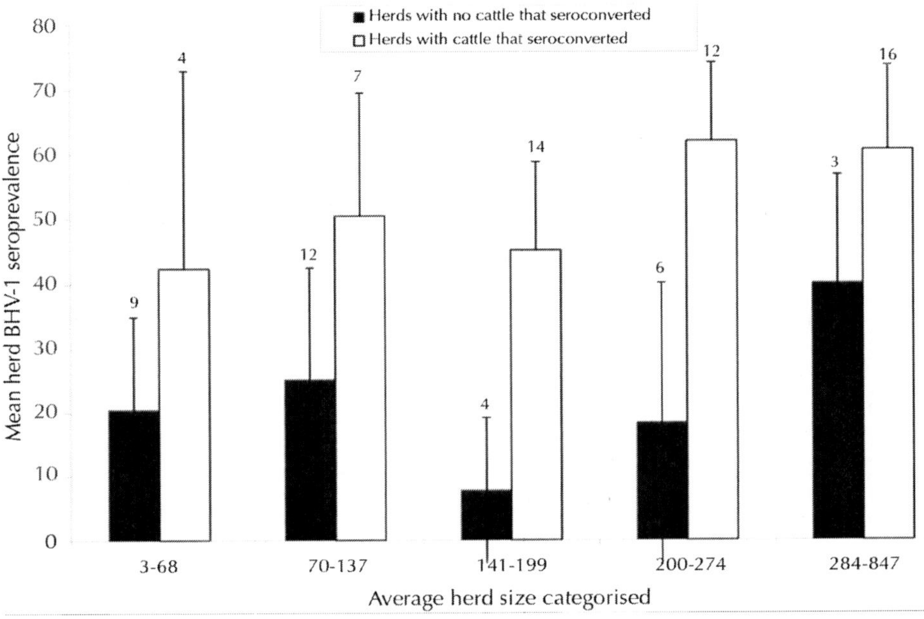

Figure 2: Mean herd BHV-1 seroprevalence and 95% CI for seropositive herds by herd size (Numbers indicate the number of herds in each category). Herds are dichotomised by presence of seroconversion.

Of the 3,452 cattle with no data on their place of birth, 2,101 (60.9%) were seropositive. Of the 10,791 cattle with data, purchased cattle were significantly more likely to be seropositive (54.1%) than homebred cattle (43.6%). The mean PP value was higher for cattle purchased into dairy herds, and increased at a greater rate over time from purchase in cattle ≥ 2 years of age at purchase (Figure 3). There was a highly significant departure from homogeneity between the four categories in Figure 3, $\chi^2 = 12137$, $P < 0.01$. There was a significant association between season of visit and PP values. Samples taken in the spring and summer had significantly lower PP values than samples taken in winter; whereas those taken in autumn had significantly higher PP values than those taken in winter.

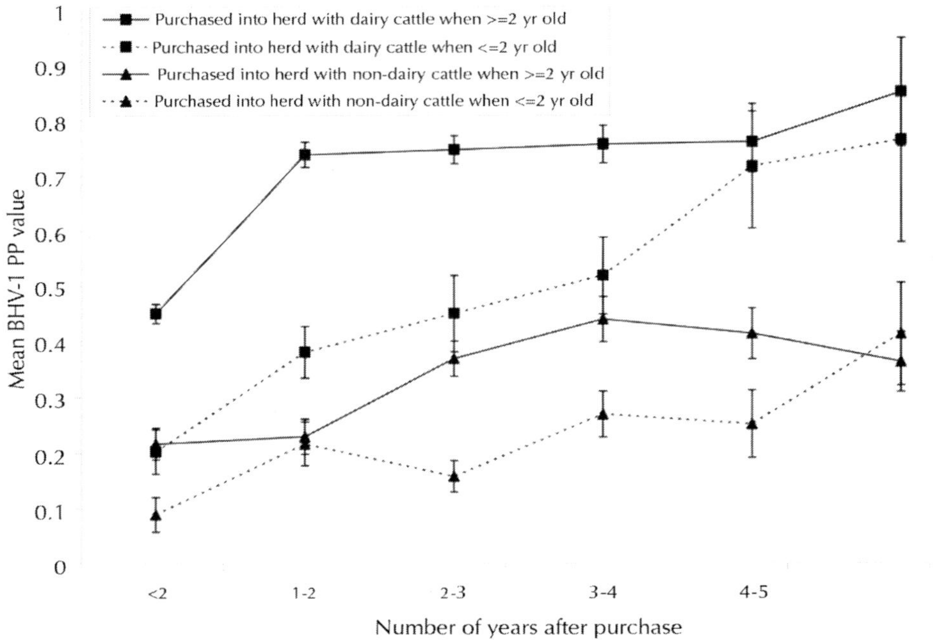

Figure 3: Mean and 95% CI BHV-1 PP value by the number of years after purchase for age group at purchase and herd purpose.

There was no significant association between restocked/ continuously stocked herds and herd seroprevalence in the univariate analysis: 16.7% of restocked herds and 16.9% continuously stocked herds had no seropositive cattle. The herd type with the highest seroprevalence was dairy cattle only (Table 3). There were no herds with dairy cattle and young stock (e.g. dairy with grower herds) that were seronegative.

Table 3: Descriptive statistics of the type of herd and number of BHV-1 sero-positive unvaccinated herds (Dataset A, see methods section)

				Cattle prevalence in positive herds		
Herd type	Mean number of cattle present in herd	No. positive herds	Total No. herds	Mean	Median	Range

Suckler herd	1–100	10	18	16.8	7.2	2.5–74.1
Suckler herd	>100	13	16	38.2	34.0	2.3–80.5
Dairy herd	1–100	5	6	27.4	17.3	7.8–58.7
Dairy herd	>100	35	36	53.1	57.7	0.5–95.4
Suckler with grower herd	1–100	4	7	44.4	49.9	2.7–75.3
Suckler with grower herd	>100	11	11	35.9	34.8	2.6–72.6
Dairy with grower herd	1–100	0	0	-	-	-
Dairy with grower herd	>100	9	9	27.2	18.6	1.9–73.0

Four herds had missing average herd size from the interview questionnaire.

Woodbine et al. BMC Veterinary Research 2009 5:5 doi:10.1186/1746-6148-5-5

Hierarchical Model Results

There were 19,633 samples (level 1), from 10,039 cattle (level 2) in 102 herds (level 3) with no missing values. In the continuous outcome model there was a significant increase in PP value with age. Cattle from herds with >200 cattle had higher PP values compared with those from herds with ≤ 200 cattle, and there were higher PP values in herds that were formed by restocking after the FMD epidemic of 2001, compared with herds that were continuously stocked. Herds with dairy cattle had higher PP values compared with those without dairy cattle. Herds with grower cattle had lower PP values compared with those without grower cattle (Table 4). In contrast to the univariate results, probably because of the relationship with the restocking variable, purchased cattle had a lower PP value than homebred cattle. The samples collected in spring and summer had significantly lower PP values than those collected in the winter, whereas those taken in the autumn had significantly higher PP values than those taken in winter. There were no significant interactions. The same fixed effects were associated with PP values in seropositive herds only (data not shown). When a variable indicating that cattle on a farm had/had not seroconverted was included (as in Figures 1 and 2) in the final model, all other variables became non-significant.

Table 4: Repeated measures multi-level model of 10,039 cattle from 102 unvaccinated herds with PP BHV-1 levels as the continuous outcome and seropositive yes/no as the discrete outcome (Dataset B, see methods section)

					Continuous			Discrete outcome		
Variable	Category level	No. herds	No. cattle	No. obs	Coef	SEb	P value	Coef	SEb	P value
Intercept					-0.05	0.08		2.95	0.42	
Triplet codea	Reactive	35	3839	7286						
	Proactive	31	4900	8660	-0.17	0.09	0.05	-0.43	0.46	0.35
	Survey	36	3665	7776	-0.10	0.09	0.28	-0.19	0.48	0.69
Restocked	No	82	10235	19398						
	Yes	24	2278	4433	0.23	0.07	<0.01	1.10	0.36	<0.01
Farm location	Area A	33	2736	4975						
	Area B	62	8644	16438	-0.01	0.09	0.91	-0.53	0.47	0.26
	Area C	11	1133	2418	-0.01	0.13	0.94	-0.51	0.72	0.48
Age (years)	2	91	1901	1969						
	3	101	3996	4401	0.08	0.01	<0.01	0.16	0.07	0.02
	4	102	3877	4325	0.24	0.01	<0.01	0.72	0.07	<0.01
	5	100	3239	3634	0.35	0.01	<0.01	1.11	0.07	<0.01
	6	101	2652	2870	0.41	0.01	<0.01	1.36	0.08	<0.01
	7	96	2011	2181	0.48	0.01	<0.01	1.51	0.08	<0.01
	8	96	1520	1658	0.53	0.02	<0.01	1.59	0.10	<0.01

	9	94	1001	1118	0.59	0.03	<0.01	1.67	0.16	<0.01
	>10	88	641	1675	0.50	0.08	<0.01	0.52	0.70	0.46
Herd size	3–68	22	644	1246						
	70–137	22	1488	2944	-0.02	0.09	0.88	-0.05	0.50	0.92
	141–199	20	2118	4232	0.05	0.09	0.59	0.88	0.49	0.07
	200–274	19	2921	5969	0.25	0.10	<0.01	1.53	0.52	<0.01
	284–847	19	5233	9331	0.40	0.10	<0.01	2.21	0.53	<0.01
Herd had	No	53	3049	6362						
dairy cattle	Yes	53	9482	17469	0.18	0.06	<0.01	1.02	0.33	<0.01
Herd had	No	79	10092	19019						
grower cattle	Yes	27	2439	4812	-0.12	0.07	<0.01	-0.29	0.35	0.41
Cattle birthplace	Homebred	83	5654	11059						
	Purchased	82	3894	7545	-0.06	0.01	0.07	-0.01	0.06	0.87
Season	Winter	55	4008	6862						
	Spring	52	4715	8166	-0.07	0.01	<0.01	-0.25	0.06	<0.01
	Summer	26	2342	3331	-0.02	0.01	0.05	-0.09	0.08	0.326
	Autumn	31	2829	4095	0.10	0.01	<0.01	0.59	0.07	<0.01

aSee Table 1 for variable definition

bStandard Error

The random effects of the repeated measures multi-level model (Variance and SE) Herd: 0.07 and 0.01; Cattle: 0.14 and 0.003; Visit: 0.08 and 0.001.

Woodbine et al. BMC Veterinary Research 2009 5:5 doi:10.1186/1746-6148-5-5

The sum of the level 1, level 2, and level 3 variances was 0.28. The greatest unexplained variance in PP values in the final multi-level model was between cattle, making up 48% of the total variance. However, the variances were significant at all three levels (Table 4).

The normal probability plots of the standardised residuals for all three levels were linear (e.g. Figure 4), indicating that the normality assumption was met. The deleted residuals did not differ greatly from the respective standardised residual values, indicating that there were no large outliers in the data at any level. When the herds, cows or samples with the largest influence were removed, the fit of the model worsened but the results of the model remained unchanged.

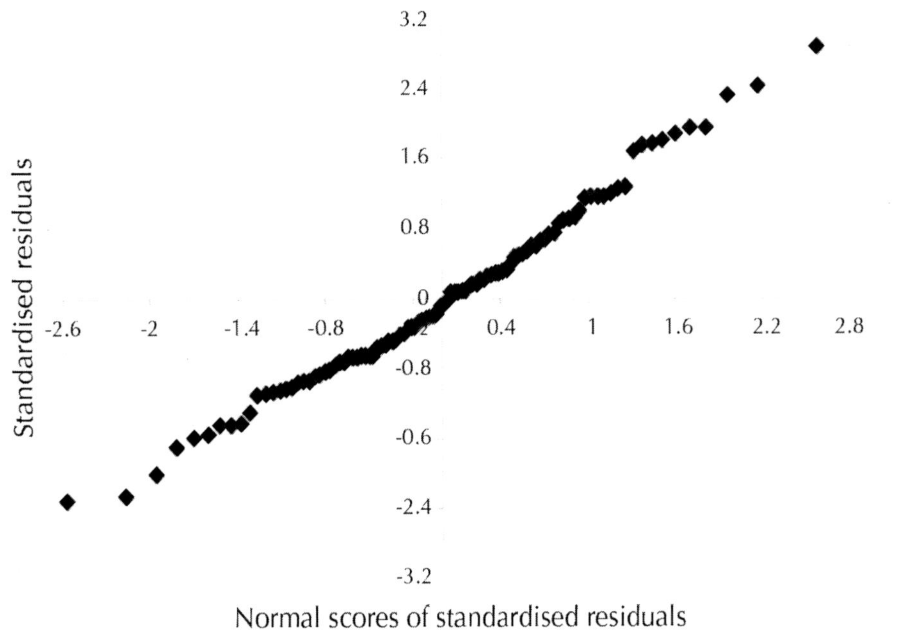

Figure 4: Normal probability plot of the standardised residuals for the herd level in Model 1 where all unvaccinated herd were included Table 3.

The estimated risks were similar when a multi-level binary logistic regression model (outcome seropositive yes/no) was fitted (Table 4). The variables that did not remain significant were whether cattle were homebred or purchased and whether herds had grower cattle.

DISCUSSION

This is the largest seroepidemiological study of BHV-1 carried out in cattle herds in the UK, and the first for more than 15 years. The seroprevalence of BHV-1 has increased dramatically since the 1960s in both cattle and herds. In the 1960s the seroprevalence in cattle was 2.1% [6], whilst in the current study, 42.5% of cattle always tested positive. Similarly, the herd prevalence was 20% in 1974 [24], and 83.2% in the current study. The differences in herd seroprevalence between the current and previous studies could be explained in part if the herds in this study were biased towards a particular location, age or cattle purpose since these were factors that influenced herd seroprevalence (Table 4). However, the consistency of seropositivity across the farms in this study over the 3 year time period suggests that infection has reached a temporal equilibrium, or possibly that seropositivity is increasing slowly.

A particularly interesting result is the higher seroprevalence in herds that were restocked after FMD. Carrique-Mas et al. (2008) [25] reported that bovine tuberculosis could be introduced into a farm at restocking when cattle were bought from herds with high incidence of infection. It is highly likely that purchase will have brought BHV-1 into restocked herds. The reason for the apparent increase in seroprevalence of BHV-1 is unknown but it might be that movement and mixing in new herds is stressful for cattle, resulting in recrudescence of virus in infected cattle that then infect susceptible cattle in the newly formed herd. In non-restocked herds, purchased cattle had a lower seroprevalence, which is contradictory to this explanation. It should also be remembered that the vaccination status of individual cattle is unknown so that the difference in seroprevalence might be explained by differences in purchasing vaccinated cattle, especially in dairy herds. There may also be complex interactions between cattle age, purchasing and restocking, since restocking of herds is very different to "routine" purchase. Additionally, the existence of multiple antigenic types (which cannot be distinguished serologically) means that interpretation of seroepidemiology is not straightforward. Whatever the cause, these results suggest that these purchased cattle were associated with a high herd seroprevalence and highlight the point that farmers should consider the antibody BHV-1 status of cattle before introduction, to prevent concomitant introduction or re-introduction of

BHV-1 of the same or a different antigenic type, that might influence disease presentation.

The seroprevalence of BHV-1 increased with herd size in the univariate analysis and in the hierarchical model; this is consistent with other studies [16,26-28]. The association with herd size was greater in herds where seroconversion occurred during the study (Figure 2), suggesting that active transmission is related positively to herd size, perhaps because larger herds have more potential transmission contacts both within the herd and with other herds (e.g. from veterinarians, other farmers and purchased cattle). However, the association between BHV-1 PP values and herd size might be confounded with other factors associated with herd size, e.g. recrudescence of infection through stress [29], or exposure to more viral types.

The age serological profile is consistent with life-long seropositivity. Antibodies to BHV-1 in calves of ≤ 6 months of age probably correspond to colostrum derived maternal immunity. This wanes by 1 year of age, and starts to rise by 2 years of age because of active infection. This suggests that the optimum age for vaccination of cattle is 10 – 14 months of age, although with some active seroconversion observed in adult cattle and a seroprevalence only exceeding 50% in older animals, vaccination is likely to have a positive impact when administered at any age. All the vaccinated herds had seropositive cattle, while approximately 80% of the unvaccinated herds had seropositive cattle. On average, less than 50% of the cattle in the unvaccinated herds tested positive at each visit, whilst >75% of the cattle from vaccinated herds were positive. These data suggest that either some cattle in vaccinated herds were not vaccinated, that vaccination does not always induce antibody or that antibody titre induced by vaccination wanes over time. It is possible that antibody titre generated by natural infection also wanes over time, but there is no previous work on this hypothesis.

In the current study, when the herd was a dairy herd rather than a suckler herd, the rate of seroconversion in adults was greater. The average age of cattle did not differ between dairy and suckler herds, and so this is a true effect, possibly due to winter housing or other stressors related to dairy cow management.

Housing and winter stressors are also an explanation for the small but significant effect of season on PP values. However, 31% and 47% of visits were 11–13 months apart for routine visits 1 and 2 and routine visits 2 and 3, respectively, so that there was a tendency for the same herds to be sampled in the same season and so herd effect is interpreted as an apparent seasonal effect. Other explanations are that seasonal culling and replacement of cattle might influence herd prevalence of BHV-1 antibodies.

All the variables above became non-significant when the binary variable seroconversion (indicating whether seroconversion was observed in the herd) was introduced into the final model. This indicates that the model risk factors are those associated with virus circulation between cattle on the farm.

The use of different modelling approaches has been discussed elsewhere [28,30] but not modelling different distributions of the same outcome. We compared these two outcomes because we wanted to investigate change in antibody level that was not necessarily occurring around the cut off. The associated risks were similar to those in Table 4 whether the data were modelled using a continuous or binary outcome, but the presence of grower cattle and purchased or homebred were not statistically significant in the binomial model, although the trends were in the same direction of risk. This suggests that these variables alter the antibody titre either always above or below the cut off and that this change was detectable in the continuous outcome model but not in the discrete model.

In the discrete model, we assumed that the serological measurement of seropositive/seronegative had perfect sensitivity and specificity. It is possible that bias could be introduced into the analysis if the sensitivity or specificity of the test varied with other variables, for example, with cattle age, or time since infection, however this has not been reported for BHV-1 antibody tests. The continuous outcome (PP) calculated from the ELISA will have had some random error (Figure 4), but avoided the need to categorise cattle as positive or negative to BHV-1 antibody, and avoided the possibility of misclassification due imperfect sensitivity and specificity, although would have retained a bias if serological measurement varied with other variables. However, the consistency between the discrete and continuous outcome models suggests that sensitivity and specificity do not alter with any of the explanatory variables in the model.

The results of this study do not necessarily represent all cattle herds in England, because of the locality of the farms sampled and because the analysis was based primarily on the serological values for BHV-1 from adult cattle. Using only unvaccinated herds in the study may have reduced the extrapolation of the results, because these herds may have had different management practices from vaccinated herds, but there were only 7 herds that reportedly used vaccination and so analysis of these herds' managements was not possible. In addition, there might have been an overestimation of the infection derived seroprevalence because purchased cattle might have been sourced from a vaccinated herd and so had antibodies derived from vaccination: we do not know the vaccination status of source herds. The serological test used in the current study did not distinguish between vaccine derived and pathogen derived antibody so this was unavoidable. It is interesting that only 7 herds were vaccinated and that farmers reported little clinical disease from BHV-1, suggesting that this infection is not an obvious production constraint or clinical disorder in most herds.

Finally, in the current analysis we could not distinguish between BHV-1 sub-types, the epidemiology of individual types might be different and this might account for some of the unexplained heterogeneity. BHV-1 subtype 3 is now classified as a new species (bovine herpesvirus-5 or BHV-5) [31]. It is probable that we were detecting antibodies to BHV-5 as well as BHV-1 because these viruses are antigenically related.

CONCLUSIONS

In conclusion, the level of BHV-1 infection has increased dramatically since previous estimates from the UK, with approximately 83% of the unvaccinated herds in the south west of England seropositive. This study adds to previous work with the finding that infection might have reached a temporal but not a spatial equilibrium and that between herd variability in PP might arise through variability in cattle age, herd size, herd purpose and the formation of new herds.

AUTHORS' CONTRIBUTIONS

KAW helped collect samples, performed the data analysis and drafted the manuscript. GFM and LEG are the funded co-applicants who designed the study, supervised data collection and analysis and finalised the manuscript. SJM coordinated and completed ELISA testing. ARV assisted in design of the questionnaire and coordinated data collection and supervised collection of blood samples. SM setup and maintained the study database and downloads. All authors read and approved the final manuscript.

ACKNOWLEDGEMENTS

We acknowledge financial support from DEFRA (SE3026) for the access to the cattle in the cohort study and BBSRC (grant number BBS/B/04854) for funding the analysis of the sera and analytical research. We are grateful for the active contribution of all the farmers, and we thank all the technicians who helped with data collection and ELISA testing.

REFERENCES

1. Wyler R, Engels M, Schwyzer M: Infectious bovine rhinotracheitis/vulvovaginitis (BHV-1). In Herpesvirus Diseases of Cattle, Horses and Pigs. Edited by Wittmann G. Kluwer Academic Publishers, Boston, Dordrecht, London; 1989:1-72.
2. Wentink GH, van Oirschot JT, Verhoef J: Risk of infection with bovine herpesvirus 1 (BHV 1): a review. Vet Q 1993, 15:30-33.
3. Bennett R, Ijpelaar J: Economic Assessment of Livestock Diseases in Great Britain. The University of Reading; 2003.
4. Ackermann M, Müller HK, Bruckner L, Kihm L: Eradication of infectious bovine rhinotracheitis in Switzerland: review and prospects. Vet Microbiol 1990, 23:365-370.
5. van Oirschot JT, Straver PJ, van Lieshout JAH, Quak J, Westenbrink F, van Exsel ACA: A subclinical infection of bulls with bovine herpesvirus type 1 at an artificial insemination centre. Vet Rec 1993, 132:32-5.
6. Dawson PS, Darbyshire JH: The occurrence and distribution in the United Kingdom of antibodies to parainfluenza 3 and infectious bovine rhinotracheitis viruses in bovine sera. Vet Rec 1964, 76:111-115.

7. Darbyshire JH, Dawson PS, Paterson AB: The isolation of infectious bovine rhinotracheitis virus in the United Kingdom: A preliminary report.
8. Vet Rec 1962, 74:156-157.
9. Dawson PS, Darbyshire JH, Loosemore RM, Paterson AB, Faull WB: Infectious bovine rhinotracheitis (IBR). A clinical condition of cattle occurring in the United Kingdom. Vet Rec 1962, 74:1379-1383.
10. Wiseman A, Msolla PM, Selman IE, Allan EM, Cornwell HJC, Pirie HM, Imray WS: An acute severe outbreak of infectious bovine rhinotracheitis: Clinical, epidemiological, microbiological and pathological aspects. Vet Rec 1978, 103:391-397.
11. Edwards S, White H, Nixon P: A study of the predominant genotypes of bovid herpesvirus 1 found in the U.K. Vet Microbiol 1990, 22:213-223.
12. Edwards S, Newman RH, White H: The virulence of British isolates of bovid herpesvirus 1 in relationship to viral genotype. Br Vet J 1991, 147:216-231.
13. Pritchard GC: Epidemiology of BHV1 infection in cattle breeding herds in Norfolk. Proceedings of the Society for Veterinary Epidemiology and Preventive Medicine, Edinburgh, 1–3 April, 1992 1992, 168-185.
14. Hogg AA: UK bovine respiratory virus serosurvey (1991/92). Proceedings of the British Cattle Veterinary Association, 1992 1992, 347-352.
15. van Wuijckhuise L, Bosch J, Franken P, Krankena K, Elbers AR: Epidemiological characteristics of bovine herpesvirus 1 infections determined by bulk milk testing of all Dutch dairy herds. Vet Rec 1998, 142:181-184.
16. van Schaik G, Dijkhuizen AA, Huirne RB, Schukken YH, Nielen M, Hage HJ: Risk factors for existence of bovine herpes virus 1 antibodies on nonvaccinating Dutch dairy farms. Prev Vet Med 1998, 34:125-136.
17. Boelaert F, Speybroeck N, de Kruif A, Aerts M, Burzykowski T, Molenberghs G, Berkvens DL: Risk factors for bovine herpesvirus-1 seropositivity. Prev Vet Med 2005, 69:285-295.

18. Faes C, Hens N, Aerts M, Shkedy Z, Geys H, Mintiens K, Laevens H, Boelaert F: Estimating herd-specific force of infection by using random-effects models for clustered binary data and monotone fractional polynomials. Appl Statist 2006, 55:595-613.
19. Bourne J: Bovine TB: The Scientific Evidence. A science base for a sustainable policy to control TB in cattle. An epidemiological investigation into bovine tuberculosis. Defra Final Report 2007.
20. Keeling MJ, Woolhouse ME, May RM, Davies G, Grenfell BT: Modelling vaccination strategies against foot-and-mouth disease. Nature 2003, 421:136-142.
21. Torstensson M: Personal communication.(Svanova) 2007.
22. Fowler J, Cohen L, Jarvis P: Practical Statistics for Field Biology. Second edition. John Wiley & Sons; 1998:166.
23. Langford IH, Lewis T: Outliers in multilevel data. J R Statist Soc A 1998, 161:121-160.
24. Rasbash J, Browne W, Goldstein H, Yang M, Plewis I, Healy M, Woodhouse G, Draper D, Langford I, Lewis T: A user's guide to MLwiN version 2.1d for use with MLwiN 1.10. Centre for Multilevel Modelling. Institute of Education, University of London; 2000.
25. Kirby FD, Martin HT, Waring MJ: A serological survey on the prevalence of infectious bovine rhinotracheitis in Buckinghamshire, Berkshire and Oxfordshire.
26. Vet Rec 1978, 103:134-136.
27. Carrique-Mas JJ, Medley GF, Green LE: Risks for bovine tuberculosis in British cattle farms restocked after the foot and mouth disease epidemic of 2001.
28. Prev Vet Med 2008, 84:85-93.
29. McDermott JJ, Kadohira M, O'Callaghan CJ, Shoukri MM: A comparison of different models for assessing variations in the sero-prevalence of infectious bovine rhinotracheitis by farm, area and district in Kenya. Prev Vet Med 1997, 32:219-34.
30. Solis-Calderon JJ, Segura-Correa VM, Segura-Correa JC, Alvarado-Islas A: Seroprevalence of and risk factors for infectious bovine rhinotracheitis in beef cattle herds of Yucatan, Mexico.
31. Prev Vet Med 2003, 57:199-208. PubMed Abstract | Publisher Full Text

32. Speybroeck N, Boelaert F, Renard D, Burzykowski T, Mintiens K, Molenberghs G, Berkvens D: Design-based analysis of surveys: a bovine herpesvirus 1 case study.
33. Epidemiol Infect 2003, 13:991-1002.
34. Enevoldsen C, Hindhede J, Kristensen T: Dairy herd management types assessed from indicators of health, reproduction, replacement, and milk production. J Dairy Sci 1996, 79:1221-36.
35. Schukken YH, Grohn YT, McDermott B, McDermott JJ: Analysis of correlated discrete observations: background, examples and solutions. Prev Vet Med 2003, 59:223-240
36. Roizman B, Desrosiers RC, Fleckenstein , Lopez C, Minson AC, Studdert MJ: The familyHerpesviridae : an update. Arch Virol 1992, 123:425-449.

Chapter 8

Risk mapping of Rinderpest sero-prevalence in Central and Southern Somalia based on spatial and network risk factors

Angel Ortiz-Pelaez[1], Dirk U Pfeiffer[1], Stefano Tempia[2], F Tom Otieno[3], Hussein H Aden[2], and Riccardo Costagli[2]

[1]Veterinary Epidemiology & Public Health Group, Department of Veterinary Clinical Sciences, The Royal Veterinary College, University of London, Hawkshead Lane, North Mymms, Hatfield, Herts, AL9 7TA, UK

[2]Terra Nuova East Africa, Raphta Road n.87 (Westlands), Maisonette 14/15, Nairobi, Kenya

[3]International Livestock Research Institute (ILRI), PO Box 30709, 00100 Nairobi, Kenya

ABSTRACT

Background

In contrast to most pastoral systems, the Somali livestock production system is oriented towards domestic trade and export with seasonal movement patterns of herds/flocks in search of water and pasture and towards export points. Data from a rinderpest survey and other data sources have been integrated to explore the topology of a contact network of cattle herds based on a spatial proximity criterion and other attributes related to cattle herd dynamics. The objective of the study is to integrate spatial mobility and other attributes with GIS and network approaches in order to develop a predictive spatial model of presence of rinderpest.

Results

A spatial logistic regression model was fitted using data for 562 point locations. It includes three statistically significant continuous-scale variables that increase the risk of rinderpest: home range radius, herd density and clustering coefficient of the node of the network whose link was established if the sum of the home ranges of every pair of nodes was equal or greater than the shortest distance between the points. The sensitivity of the model is 85.1% and the specificity 84.6%, correctly classifying 84.7% of the observations. The spatial autocorrelation not accounted for by the model is negligible and visual assessment of a semivariogram of the residuals indicated that there was no undue amount of spatial autocorrelation. The predictive model was applied to a set of 6176 point locations covering the study area. Areas at high risk of having serological evidence of rinderpest are located mainly in the coastal districts of Lower and Middle Juba, the coastal area of Lower Shabele and in the regions of Middle Shabele and Bay. There are also isolated spots of high risk along the border with Kenya and the southern area of the border with Ethiopia.

Conclusions

The identification of point locations and areas with high risk of presence of rinderpest and their spatial visualization as a risk map will be useful for informing the prioritization of disease surveillance and control activities for rinderpest in Somalia. The methodology applied here, involving spatial and network parameters, could also be applied to other diseases and/or species as part of a standardized approach for the design of risk-based surveillance activities in nomadic pastoral settings.

BACKGROUND

Somalia's livestock production sector accounts for at least 40% of the gross domestic product (GDP) with 55% of the human population being directly involved in the rearing of livestock [1]. Pastoral movements across Somalia's borders for the purposes of grazing livestock and livestock-related trade have occurred for centuries [2], resulting in seasonal movement patterns of herds/flocks in search of water and pasture. Moreover, in contrast to most pastoral systems, which are normally aimed at household subsistence, the Somali livestock production system is oriented towards domestic trade and export [3]. Livestock are shipped to various countries in the Arabian Peninsula, and trekked or transported to markets in Kenya, Djibouti, and Ethiopia [4]. In 2007 some 1,639,625 heads of cattle, sheep, goats and camels were exported through Bossasso port and a total of 1,633,793 through Berbera port [4], the two major export markets in the country.

Despite the collapse of the Somali government in 1991 and the lack of continued delivery of public services, an informal system of stateless order, social trust and an informal economy have allowed rural and urban populations to survive unfavourable economic and political circumstances [5]. But the Somali livestock industry is therefore now even more vulnerable to the introduction of bans by importing countries for two reasons. One being the stringent measures for livestock trade specified under the Sanitary and Phytosanitary (SPS) Agreement of the World Trade Organizationhttp://www.wto.org *webcite*, of which Somalia is not a member, and the other the poor standards of veterinary services and the absence of control measures for fighting trans-boundary animal diseases. The high mobility of the livestock population poses an additional challenge for the control and establishment of credible certification systems for the major trans-boundary diseases occurring in Somalia. An understanding of the aggregation/dispersion mechanisms and contact structure of the Somali livestock potentially could assist in setting up appropriate spatial risk-based surveillance activities and control measures that may lead to the establishment of an internationally accepted certification system for this nomadic pastoral livestock production system.

Data on the geographical patterns of human and animal population distributions are now commonly considered in epidemiological studies. High density of susceptible populations has been shown to be a key factor in the transmission of infectious diseases in humans [6]. In the case of animal populations, spatial proximity is closely linked to the transmission of many infectious diseases [7]. The geo-referencing of animals kept in herds through the point location of the farm is relatively simple and cost-effective [8]. However in settings where mobility is a major feature of the husbandry systems the geographical location of animals is no longer a discrete entity hence alternative approaches are required for the collection and analysis of their spatial data.

Network data are not usually linked to geographical data, and social network analysis rarely considers the spatial configuration of the links [9] apart from the pure visualization of the networks. Definitions of links within networks based on spatial criteria such as the distance between pairs of nodes, usually estimated using the Euclidean distance ("as the crow flies") are rarely available in the literature. For example, Webb [10] made the assumption in her analysis that there was a link between two farms if their postcodes were less than 25 km apart, as a proxy for the catchment area of farm animal veterinary practices. Dent et al. [11] considered poultry premises to be linked if they were within 3 km distance from each other.

The purpose of epidemiological modelling of spatial data is to explain or predict the occurrence of disease [12-18]. The production of risk maps can guide decision makers provided that the underlying assumptions of uncertainty and variability are exposed [19]. Using the data from a previous rinderpest survey conducted in the Central and Southern regions of Somalia, it was possible to explore the topology of a contact network of cattle herds based on a spatial proximity criterion and other attributes related to cattle herd dynamics. The objective of the current study is to integrate spatial mobility and other attributes with GIS and network approaches in order to investigate their effect on disease presence and develop a predictive spatial model of presence of rinderpest. The risk map generated by the predictive model can be used to inform the design of risk-based surveillance activities of rinderpest by identifying high-risk point locations where to prioritize disease surveillance and control activities. Surveillance efforts could be targeted at high-risk areas which would lead to more effective use of the scarce veterinary resources in Somalia, and ultimately, contribute to the establishment of an internationally credible certification system for livestock export by nomadic pastoral systems. The standardisation of the proposed methodology for cattle will serve as a model for other livestock species (e.g. small ruminants and camelids) and other diseases.

METHODS

Rinderpest data

A cross-sectional survey was carried out in Central and Southern Somalia to estimate the prevalence of rinderpest (RP) in 2002-2003. The study area covered ten administrative regions of Central and Southern Somalia: Mudug, Galgadud, Hiran, Middle Shabele, Lower Shabele, Bay, Bakool, Lower Juba, Middle Juba and Gedo (Figure 1). Ninety percent of Somalia's cattle population are kept in these regions [20]. Details of the design and implementation of the survey are described elsewhere [21].

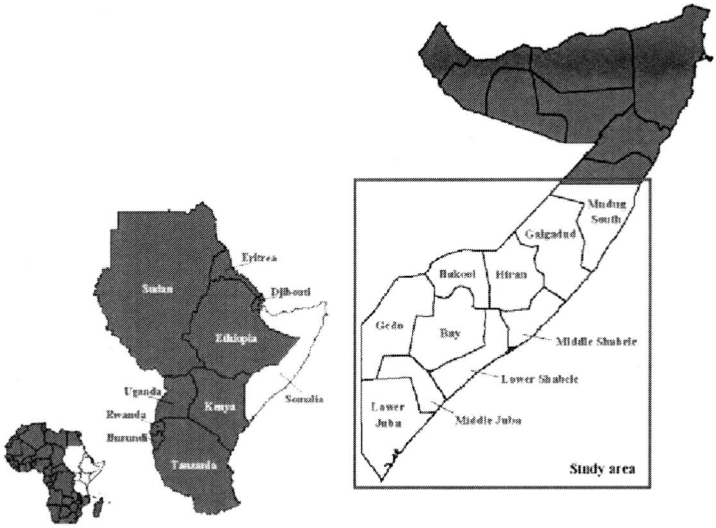

Figure 1: Map of Somalia with the names of the Central and Southern regions included in the study area.

At selected sampling sites, a minimum number of 15 eligible animals were sampled per herd and questionnaires were administered to the livestock owners of the sampled herds in order to collect data on species, herd/flock size and location during each climatic season over the two years prior to the date the survey was conducted in that point and livestock markets (primary and secondary) where the pastoralists sold their animals during the same period. A total of 9216 serum samples were collected from cattle aged 1 to 3 years at 562 sampling sites. In addition, 1071 sera were collected from cattle older than 3 years at 58 sampling sites. All serum samples collected were tested for the presence of RP antibodies using a RP Competitive Enzyme Linked Immunosorbent Assay (C-ELISA) directed against the H protein of the virus [22]. All samples having a percentage of inhibition (PI) above 50% were considered positive in accordance with the OIE recommendation for testing large numbers of sera.

Home range

The home-range (Hr) of the 562 point locations where at least one cattle herd was located was estimated by first obtaining the geographical coordinates [23,24] for each of the points where the herd/s had been reported during the surveyed seasons (Jiilaal: Dec. - Mar.; Gu': Apr. - Jun.; Xagaa: Jul. - Sep. Dayr: Oct. - Nov.) over the two years prior to the time of the survey. If a particular location was not included in the available databases then the location was visited and the geographical coordinates were recorded. The home range for each point was then calculated based on these point locations using the minimum convex polygon (MCP) method [25] and adding a buffer of 5 km around the MCP in order to account for the daily mobility of the herds. The area (in km2) of the MCP represents the estimated home range for a particular point based on the observed movements of the herd/s in that point. Figure 2 displays the location of a subset of locations for a herd and the resulting MCP polygon from which a circular home range was calculated.

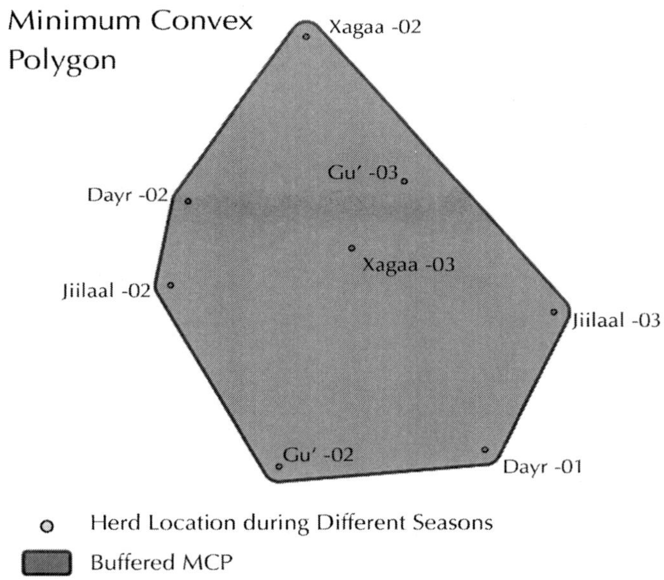

Figure 2: Example for the calculation of the home-range using the Minimum Convex Polygon (MCP) method for one of the point locations of the Rinderpest survey.

A map representing the spatial variation in home range area (km^2) for cattle herds was then generated using kriging techniques [26-29]. Kriging is a group of geostatistical techniques for interpolating the value of a random field at an unobserved location based on observed values at nearby locations [28]. The home range values (z) for each point included in the study were used to generate the kriged surface utilizing as location the coordinates (x, y) of the centroid of the home-range polygon estimated for each individual herd. The kriged surface representing the average home range estimates at each location was created by first fitting an nth order polynomial surface to the data [30]. Akaike's Information Criteria (AIC) was used to compare the fit of the different surfaces from 1st to 4th polynomial order and different covariance functions (Gaussian, exponential, spherical and Matern) [31]. Then, the covariance structure of the data was modelled using a exponential covariance function with a range value of $\theta = 0.24$ and a nugget of $\alpha = 0.35$. The final surface was generated by kriging the residuals of the surface using the selected exponential covariance function. The kriged map of the spatial pattern of average cattle home range is displayed in Figure 3.

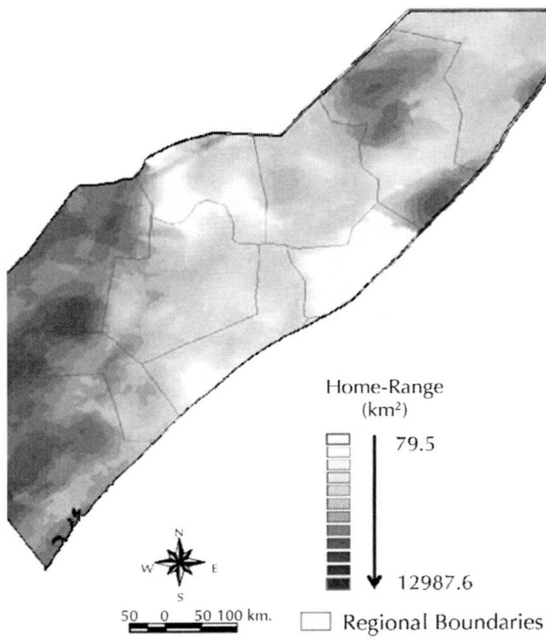

Figure 3: Cattle home range distribution map of the study area obtained via the kriging method.

Attributes for the 562 point locations were generated through spatial queries and analysis in ArcGIS 9.2. (© ESRI), using as unique identifier a point location reference number linked to the projected coordinates. Seven attributes were extracted for each point location. (1) The type of point (categorical): villages, towns [24], water points [23], primary/secondary markets [32], and grazing points [33]. (2) Proximity to roads (binary): less than 500 meters from a main road. (3) Proximity to trade routes (binary): the locations of three major trade routes were recorded in southern and central Somalia by Terra Nuova [32] by use of a radio collar GPS fitted to an animal within the traded herds being trekked from secondary markets to export points. The proximity was based on whether a point's estimated home range as described above intersected the trade routes. (4) Speed at trade route (numeric): the speed of the movement at each trade route point was calculated for segments of time and distance between points along the trade routes derived from the spatial join of collar (cattle) and drover (handler) GPS data and then aggregated based on drover GPS locations. If the point was linked to a trade route, speed in km/h was included. (5) Home range radius (numeric): radius of the home range assuming circular shape (method described above). (6) Herd density (numeric): herd density values assigned to the survey points through intersection of the points with a distribution map of herd density generated through moving average neighbourhood analysis [31] from livestock census data [20]. (7) Herd size (numeric): herd size values assigned to the survey points through intersection of the points with a distribution map of herd sizes [21].

Network

The contact network between nomadic herds was constructed using the 6738 point locations of towns, villages, watering points and grazing areas, including the 562 points from the survey, extracted from the above-mentioned databases. The home range for each of the 6738 points was assigned by spatially overlaying the point location map with the interpolated home range map shown in Figure 3. Once all points had been assigned a home range, home radii were calculated assuming a circular shape for the home ranges. Thereafter a Euclidean distance matrix between each pair of points was generated using the Hawth's Analysis Tool for ArcGIShttp://www.spatialecology.

com/htools/ *webcite*. If the distance between a pair of points was less than the sum of their home range radii then these two points were linked by a symmetric unvalued link. Thus the links between nodes in the network were derived from contact (Points d and e in Figure 4) or overlap of the points' home ranges (Points b and c in Figure 4). A graphic representation of the comparison of home range radii and distances between points to generate the network is illustrated in Figure 4. The following general parameters of the symmetric binary network were extracted: number of nodes, number of links, density, giant weak component and average distance among reachable pairs. For individual nodes, the following centrality measures were extracted: degree, betweenness, closeness and clustering coefficient.

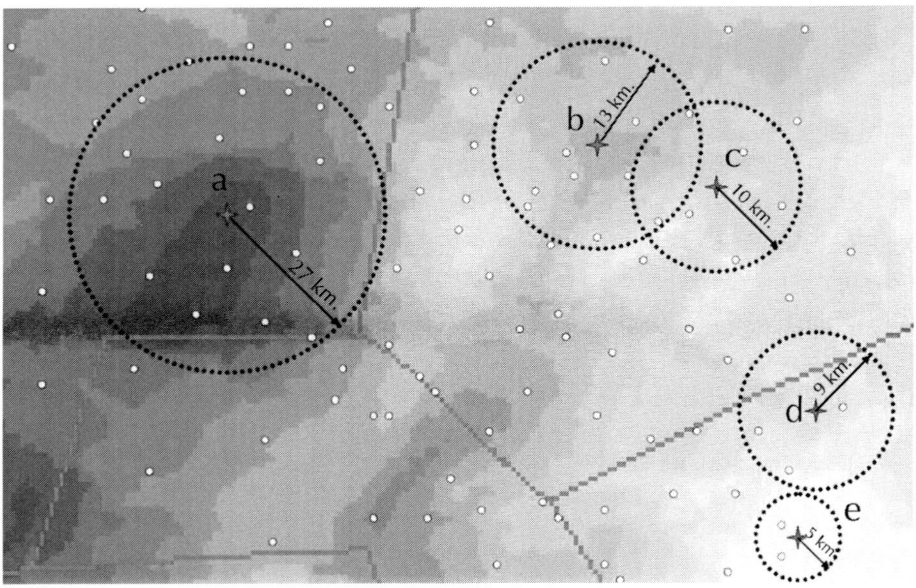

Figure 4: Graphical representation of the process used for generating the herd movement contact network. Points b and c and d and e are linked. Point a is not linked to b, c, d or e.

Spatial logistic model

The study population comprised the initial 562 randomly selected locations included in the cross-sectional rinderpest survey, for which data on number of animals sampled and test results were available. If we consider the number of positive samples for Rinderpest at point i out of N_i sampled animals, Y_i is a binomial random variable Y_i ~Bin (N_i, p_i) with pi being the prevalence of infection at each point. The spatial binomial logistic model is given by:

$$\log\left(\frac{p_i}{1-p_i}\right) = \beta_0 + \beta_i x_i + S_i + \xi_i$$

where β_0 is the intercept, x_i the covariates, β_i the regression coefficients, ξ_i normally distributed non-correlated residuals and Si the spatial component (spatial autoregressive coefficient), which is assumed to have zero mean, variance σ^2 and an isotropic covariance function ρ (d_{ij} θ), where θ is the range coefficient and measures the decay of the spatial autocorrelation and d_{ij} is the Euclidean distance between each pair of points.

A generalized linear mixed model with a logit link function was fitted. The outcome variable was the count of rinderpest positive samples expressed as a binomial distribution to account for the variation in the number of animals tested. The following covariates were introduced in the multivariable model as fixed effects: type of point, next to road, linked to trade route, speed at trade route, herd density, herd size, home range radius, degree, betweenness, closeness, inclusion in the giant weak component and clustering coefficient. An exponential spatial covariance structure (exp ($-d_{ij}/\theta$)) was included as a random effect. The analysis was implemented using restricted pseudo likelihood with the GLIMMIX procedure of SAS 9.1 (© 2002-2003 by SAS Institute Inc., Cary, NC, USA). Linearity of the effects was tested by categorising continuous variables into three-category variables. The statistical significance of the fixed effect variables was determined using Type III tests. The ability of the binomial model to predict the outcome was estimated using as cut-off point the mean of the fitted probabilities predicted by the model in order to transform them into a binary outcome [34]. Predicted probabilities below the cut-off value were considered as predicting absence (0) and probabilities above the cut-off value were considered predicting presence (1).

Once the final model was fitted, a semivariogram of the residuals was generated using the ArcGIS 9.2 Geostatistical Analyst extension (© ESRI) for assessing the potential presence of spatial autocorrelation in the model residuals. The logistic regression model equation was applied to the set of 6176 point locations using their specific covariate patterns. Attributes for the significant variables of the final model were extracted for the set of point locations using the same methods as for the survey points. The predicted prevalence using the final model equation for each point location was exported to ArcGIS 9.2 (© ESRI) for visualization of the resulting risk map. A kernel smoothed intensity map was produced with 50 km bandwidth and 5 km grid cells using the Spatial Analyst extension of ArcGIS 9.2 (© ESRI).

RESULTS

The 562 point locations included in the survey consisted of 479 villages (85.3%), 6 towns (1%) and 77 grazing points (13.7%). Fifty-five of the points were linked to at least one of the three trade routes (9.8%). The average size of the home range radii was 23 km (STD: 13.8 Range: 0-97 km). The average herd density across the points was 13.3 herds (STD: 6.5 Range: 4-24) and the average herd size was 45.6 (STD: 27.5 Range: 10.4-164.5). The number of point locations with rinderpest confirmed in at least one of the animals sampled was 206 (36.6%) with a mean prevalence among positive points of 18.2% (Range: 0.18-82.4%). The distribution of the point locations of the rinderpest survey and their disease status are displayed in Figure 5.

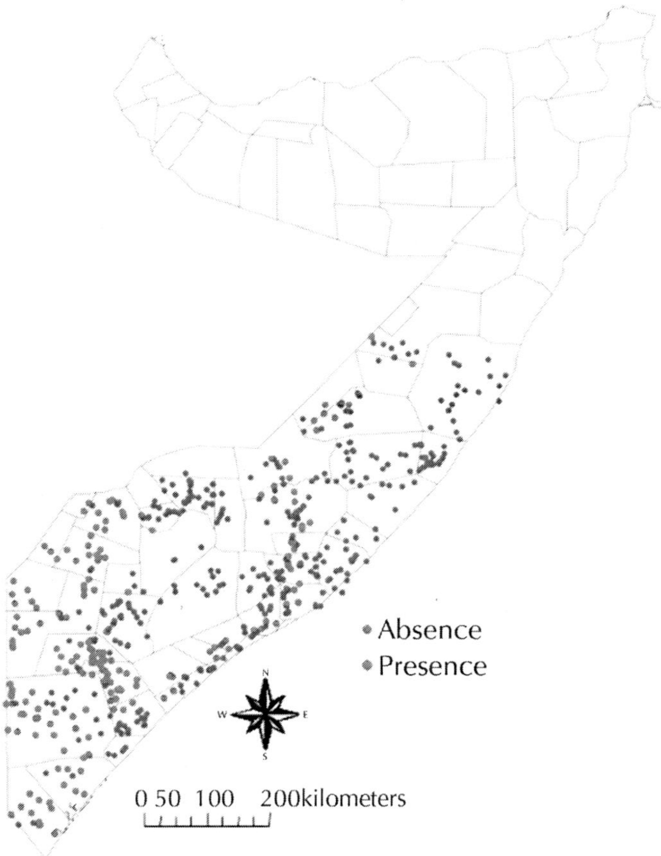

Figure 5: Distribution of the 562 point locations of the rinderpest survey and their serological status (Presence/Absence).

The final model was fitted using data for 562 point locations and contains three continuous-scale variables significant at $P < 0.05$ level: home range radius, herd density and clustering coefficient. The regression coefficients of the model, their standard errors, P values and the corresponding odds ratios with 95% confidence intervals are shown in Table 1. An increase of 1 km in the home range radius increases the risk of having rinderpest by 1.6%. For an increase of one herd in the herd density at a point location the risk of having rinderpest increases by 12%. The risk of serological evidence of rinderpest being present amongst the animal sampled at a point location with maximum clustering coefficient (1) is nearly 20 times the risk of a point whose linked points are not connected with each other. All Type III effects for the variables included in the final model were significant at $P < 0.05$ level. Predicted prevalence for each point location was converted into a dichotomous presence/absence outcome using the mean of the fitted continuous-scale probability values as the cut-off; predicted probabilities less than 0.126 were classified as absence of rinderpest and those greater than 0.126 were classified as presence of rinderpest. The sensitivity of the model is 85.1% and the specificity 84.6%, correctly classifying 84.7% of the observations. Table 2 shows the comparison between fitted and observed values.

Table 1: Coefficients of the final binomial generalized mixed model (GLM) with standard errors, odds ratios and 95% confidence intervals

	Coefficient	Standard Error	P-value	Odds Ratio (95% CI)
Intercept	-7.28	0.68	P < 0.001	
Home range radius (in Km)	0.016	0.004	P < 0.001	1.016 (1.008-1.025)
Herd density	0.11	0.02	P < 0.001	1.12 (1.06-1.18)
Clustering coefficient (cc1)	2.97	0.72	P < 0.001	19.6 (4.7-81.8)

Ortiz-Pelaez *et al. BMC Veterinary Research* 2010 **6**:22 , doi:10.1186/1746-6148-6-22

Table 2: Predicted outcomes from the final binomial generalized mixed model (GLM) compared to the observed data

		Observed		
		Presence	Absence	Total
Predicted*	Presence	80	72	152
	Absence	14	396	410
	Total	94	468	562

*Presence: if the observed prevalence or the predicted probability are greater than the mean of the distribution of the fitted probabilities of the model. Absence if they are lower

Ortiz-Pelaez *et al.* *BMC Veterinary Research* 2010 **6**:22 , doi:10.1186/1746-6148-6-22

The variance of the underlying residual spatial effect is 0.003, and the distance at which the correlation between point locations has decreased to the 0.05 level is 1.5 km. Visual inspection of the semivariogram of the model residuals as displayed in Figure 6 suggests the absence of spatial autocorrelation.

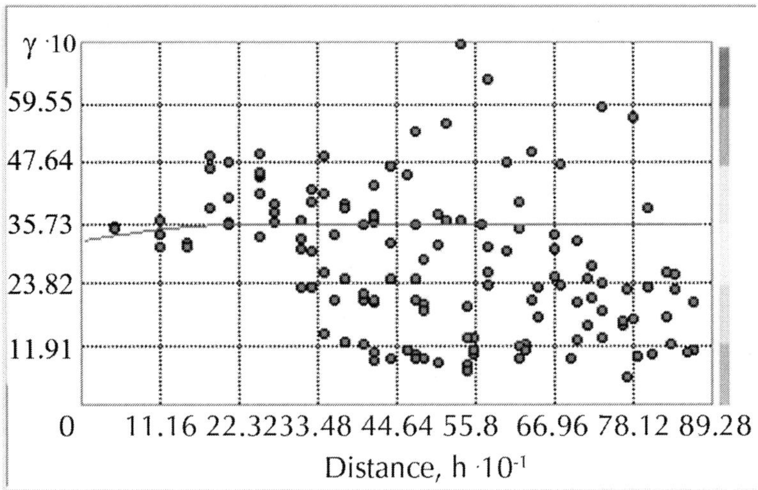

Figure 6: Semivariogram of the residuals of the final binomial GLM model. X axis: distance of the space intervals (h). Y axis: semivariance (γ)

The network contains 6738 nodes and 319,887 links with a density of 1.4% and an average degree of 224.68 (range: 1-605). The average distance between reachable pairs is 7.7 links with the maximum distance between two points being 24. There is a giant weak component containing 2950 nodes (43.78%). Within the network the 562 points of the survey had an average degree of 169 (STD: 118 Range: 2-605), average betweenness of 0.001 (STD: 0.004 Range: 0-0.05), average closeness of 0.12 (STD: 0.023 Range: 0.08-0.17) and average clustering coefficient 0.67 (STD: 0.01 Range: 0.3-1).

The risk map for the 6176 point locations is shown in Figure 7. Predicted prevalence of rinderpest has been aggregated into four categories for visual display in different colours: <4%, 4-10%, >10-20% and >20%. The kernel smoothed intensity map in Figure 8 shows predicted prevalence using 5 km square grid cells. Assuming the equivalence of predicted prevalence and probability of presence of rinderpest, the areas at high risk of having serological evidence of rinderpest amongst the animals sampled, as predicted by the model, are located mainly in the south of the study area, in the coastal districts of Lower and Middle Juba, the coastal area of Lower Shabele and in the regions of Middle Shabele and Bay. There are also isolated spots of high risk along the border with Kenya and the southern area of the border with Ethiopia. Very low risk areas are situated in the central and northern regions of the study areas, in the regions of Galgadud and Mudug, with low risk areas in the regions of Bay, Gedo and both inland Middle and Lower Shabele.

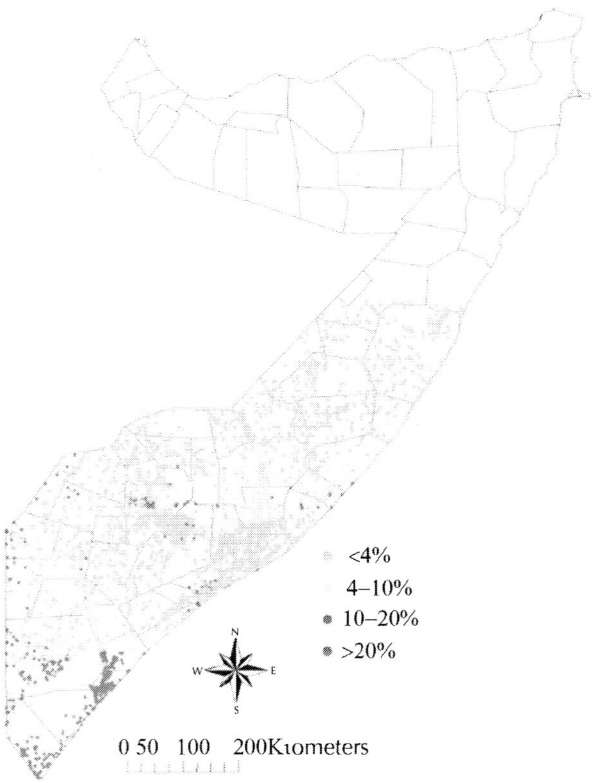

Figure 7: Risk map of the 6176 point locations in the study area based on the probability of Rinderpest presence according to the predictive model.

Evaluating the model by comparing the predicted high-risk areas as shown in the point location map (Figure 7) and the kernel smoothed intensity risk map (Figure 8) with the findings of the rinderpest survey (Figure 5), the model appears to correctly predict the presence of rinderpest in Lower and Middle Juba and Middle Shabele. The model predicts Gedo and Western Galgadu on the border of Ethiopia as low risk, both of which are provinces where rinderpest was confirmed during the survey. On the other hand, the model predicts high risk at point locations in areas where the survey did not find positive cases, such as the border area between Bakool and Bay. It is worth stressing the difference in the scale of risk between the risk point location and the kernel smoothed intensity map where the colour grade in the latter determines the risk for 25 km^2 raster cell areas at much lower scale than the point map.

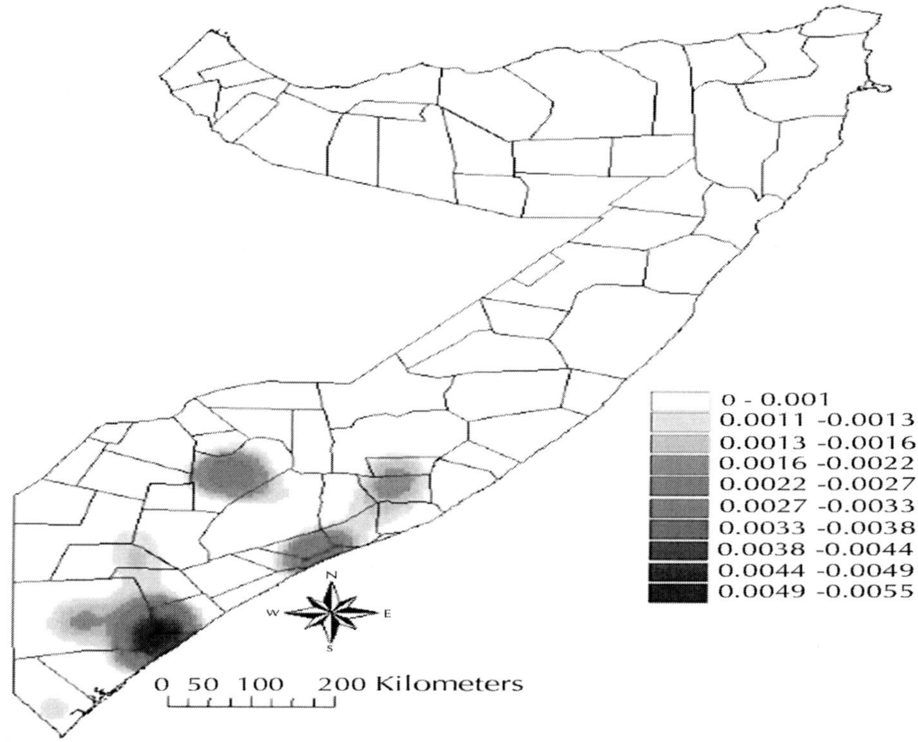

Figure 8: Kernel smoothed intensity map of the predicted probability of Rinderpest presence according to the predictive model (5 km grid cells, 50 km bandwidth).

DISCUSSION

This study has applied spatial and network analysis techniques to a combination of observed and estimated data with the objective to produce a predictive model for the presence of serological evidence of rinderpest in the southern and central regions of Somalia. Incorporating the network framework into GIS has been attempted before mainly in geography and social sciences. For example, Faust et al. [9] showed how social relations can be determined by geographical location and other spatially-related attributes. In the context of disease transmission, Rothenberg et al. [6] demonstrated that social and geographical distance can support transmission of disease. Following the same rationale the main hypothesis tested in this study was whether the presence of rinderpest is associated with the network centrality related to its geographical location and/or to other attributes of the geographical locations. The results have shown the significance of both types of factors. One of these is the degree of interactions between herds due to overlapping home ranges in neighbouring areas, expressed by the clustering coefficient of the nodes derived from the spatial contact network. The other is the home range radius or area where nomadic herds graze throughout the year and the herd density are both significant risk factors. The combination of the three significant factors reveals the importance for the presence of rinderpest of local neighbourhood and geographic compactness interacting in densely populated areas, an effect that has been reported before for human diseases such as STDs and HIV-AIDS [35,6].

Network parameters that take into account paths between all possible pairs of nodes such as betweenness and closeness did not appear to be significantly associated with the presence of disease. Large intermediaries or globally relevant nodes in the network represented by high betweenness and closeness are not roles that increase the risk of disease presence in the population of the survey, nor is the membership in within-network structures such as the giant weak component. Although two nodes/points far apart can be linked via a path of overlapping home ranges, being reachable by many other nodes in the network, in between many other shorter paths, or included in a connected subpopulation of nodes, the results suggest that the amount of overlap between neighbouring herd home ranges is the only network feature that substantially increases the risk of rinderpest. The spread of rinderpest to distant areas may follow other paths unaccounted for in this study. For example, the effect of markets has not been addressed in this analysis. It would be advised to investigate additional potential risk factors such as presence of or distance to local or regional markets. Nor has the possible risk attributed to long-distance movements via trade routes been assessed given the presence in the dataset of only three trade routes linked to each other and located in the southern districts of the study area. Incorporating more comprehensive data on putative risk factors such as the movement of the herds to markets and borders with neighbouring countries would allow testing these hypotheses.

The inclusion of variables with a strong spatial component in the multivariable analysis required the application of an analytical method that could account for the dependence of the network data due to both the inherent nature of the network data and the spatial definition of the link. Thus, the general assumption of dependence within the network data analyzed is confirmed by both the network parameterization and the spatial nature of the link. In fact, the spatial component of the binomial generalized linear mixed model, the spatial autoregressive coefficient, is similar to the local and interaction effects in network models [36] in what Anselin [37] called the family of autocorrelation models. In both cases the specifications of the chosen weight matrix are important for testing the statistical significance of a particular parameter. In this case, the spatial correlation function accounts at the same time for the similarity of home range radius and herd density between proximal points and the similarity of clustering coefficient of points linked in the network.

The internal validation of the final model showed a very high predictive ability. Its application to a different dataset has produced risk maps of point locations and areas based on the model estimates. In general, the location of the high-risk points agrees with the observed points positive to rinderpest in the original dataset, which suggests that the areas affected by rinderpest are characterised by large home ranges, large herd density and strong local interaction between neighbouring nomadic herds. However there is an area in Gedo region close to the border with Ethiopia and Somalia where the risk map predicts points of high prevalence whereas the kernel smoothed intensity map does not. This is due to the presence in that area of a small number of points with very large home ranges and high herd density that increase the risk at point level but dilute the risk at area level. This is a methodological constraint rather than an incoherent result given the difficulty of obtaining stable risk estimates if intensities vary substantially across an area[7].

Both, the point and area risk maps, identified a high risk area that the survey sampled at low intensity and did not detect rinderpest. It is located in the northern part of the Bay region close to the border with Bakool. These areas of predicted high risk and for which disease data is sparse or absent and were not well covered by the survey should therefore be prioritised for surveillance purposes.

The risk maps have identified areas in the Central and Southern regions of Somalia where veterinary authorities should concentrate their efforts for implementation of surveillance activities. It is recommended to validate these results with local experts and through further surveys to ascertain the rinderpest status in areas of predicted high risk where the disease is not currently known to be present. In this respect similar serological studies subsequently conducted in the study area detected rinderpest antibodies in the high-risk areas identified under this study. However, the observed sero-prevalence in these areas was observed to decline over time [38-40]. Similar sero-prevalence studies conducted in neighbouring areas of Kenya and Ethiopia in subsequent years also showed a very low sero-prevalence or the absence of rinderpest antibodies[41]. The progressive decline in rinderpest antibody prevalence is consistent with virus extinction. The verification of freedom from infection from the Somali Eco-System is currently in progress.

This methodology can also be used for other diseases and/or species as part of a standardized approach for the design of risk-based surveillance activities in nomadic pastoral settings. The detection of high risk areas and hot spots will assist veterinary authorities in strengthening the veterinary surveillance in such areas in order to apply control measures at the local level and to minimize the potential spread of the disease to other regions. The application of disease control measures based on geographical factors and applied at local/ compartmental level could be a starting point for the establishment of an internationally recognised certification system in settings where large-scale surveillance and control activities cannot be implemented.

CONCLUSIONS

This study demonstrates the potential for the integration of different data sources and analytical methods for the development of a spatial and network predictive model of the presence of rinderpest in central and southern Somalia. The identification of point locations and areas with high risk of presence of rinderpest and their spatial visualization as a risk map can assist in prioritizing disease surveillance and control activities for rinderpest in Somalia.

Although considerable progress on RP eradication has been achieved in the study area since this study was conducted, the value and application of the applied methodology remains of interest for the investigation of livestock diseases in nomadic and semi-nomadic pastoral systems. This methodology can be used as part of a standardized approach for developing new decision-support tools for the design of risk-based surveillance activities in nomadic pastoral settings where the particular husbandry system, the lack of infrastructure and the inadequacy of the available veterinary services prevent the implementation of comprehensive control policies.

AUTHORS' CONTRIBUTIONS

AOP designed the study, conducted the network and multivariable statistical analysis and wrote the manuscript. DUP conducted the multivariable statistical analysis and reviewed the manuscript. ST conducted the rinderpest survey, designed the study and conducted the analysis of estimation of home range. FTO collected and managed data and reviewed the manuscript. HHA conducted the rinderpest survey and RC reviewed the manuscript. All authors read and approved the final manuscript.

ACKNOWLEDGEMENTS

The paper originates from activities carried out within the frame of the "Improvement and Diversification of Somali Livestock Trade and Marketing", project funded by the EC and Royal Danish Embassy and implemented by Terra Nuova and ILRI.

The content of this publication is the sole responsibility of the authors and in no way reflects the views of the European Union or/and the Royal Danish Embassy.

REFERENCES

1. Food and Agriculture Organization (FAO): *Somalia, towards a livestock sector strategy. Final Report.* FAO-World Bank Cooperative Programme. European Union; 2004. Report No.: 04/001 IC-SOM
2. Lindley A: *Somalia Country Study. A part of the report on Informal Remittance Systems in Africa, Caribbean and Pacific (ACP) countries (Ref: RO2CS008).* ESRC Centre on Migration, Policy and Society (COMPAS). Oxford, UK; 2005.
3. Abdullahi AM: Pastoral Production Systems in Africa. A Study of Nomadic Household Economy and Livestock Marketing in Central Somalia. In *Farming Systems and Resource Economics in the Tropics (Germany). Volume 8.* Wissenschaftsverlag Vauk. Kiel (Germany); 1990::266.
4. Food Security Analysis Unit (FSAU): Livestock export data for Somalia. Food Security Analysis Unit-Somalia, Food and Agriculture Organization.[http://www.fsausomali.org/fileadmin/uploads/1273_01.pdf] 2008.
5. Little PD: *Somalia: Economy Without State.* Bloomington and Indianapolis: Indiana University Press; 2003:206.
6. Rothenberg R, Muth SQ, Malone S, Potterat JJ, Woodhouse DE: Social and geographic distance in HIV risk. *Sex Transm Dis* 2005, 32(8):506-12.
7. Pfeiffer DU, Robinson TP, Stevenson M, Stevens K, Rogers DJ, Clements ACA: *Spatial Analysis in Epidemiology.* Oxford University Press. Oxford, UK; 2008:142.
8. Durr PA, Froggatt AEA: How best to geo-reference farms? A case study from Cornwall, England. *Prev Vet Med* 2002, 56(1):51-62.
9. Faust K, Entwistel B, Rindfuss RR, Walsh SJ, Sawangdee Y: Spatial arrangements of social and economic networks among villages in Nang Rong District, Thailand. *Social Networks* 1999, 21:311-337.

10. Webb CR: Farm animal networks: unravelling the contact structure of the British sheep population. *Prev Vet Med* 2005, 68(1):3-17.

11. Dent JE, Kao RR, Kiss IZ, Hyder K, Arnold M: Contact structures in the poultry industry in Great Britain: Exploring transmission routes for a potential avian influenza virus epidemic. *BMC Veterinary Research* 2008, 4:27.

12. Pfeiffer DU, Duchateau L, Kruska RL, Ushewokunze-Obatolu U, Perry BD: A spatially predictive logistic regression model for occurrence of theileriosis outbreaks in Zimbabwe. *Epidemiologie et santé animale* 1997., 31-32 1212.1-3.

13. Baylis M, Mellor PS, Wittman EJ, Rogers DJ: Prediction of areas around the Mediterranean at risk of bluetongue by modelling the distribution of its vector using satellite imaging. *The Veterinary Record* 2001, 149:639-643.

14. McKenzie JS, Morris RS, Pfeiffer DU, Dymond JR: Application of remote sensing to enhance the control of wildlife-associated Mycobacterium bovis infection. *PE&RS - Photogrammetric Engineering & Remote Sensing* 2002, 68(2):153-159.

15. Tum S, Puotinen ML, Copeman DB: A geographic information systems model for mapping risk of fasciolosis in cattle and buffaloes in Cambodia. *Veterinary Parasitology* 2004, 122:141-149.

16. Pfeiffer DU, Minh PQ, Martin V, Epprecht M, Otte MJ: An analysis of the spatial and temporal patterns of highly pathogenic avian influenza occurrence in Vietnam using national surveillance data. *The Veterinary Journal* 2007, 174:302-309.

17. Gilbert M, Xiao X, Pfeiffer DU, Epprecht M, Boles S, Czarnecki C, Chaitaweesub P, Kalpravidh W, Minh PQ, Otte MJ, Martin V, Slingenbergh J: Mapping H5N1 highly pathogenic avian influenza risk in Southeast Asia. *PNAS March 25* 2008, 105(12):4769-4774.

18. Boender GJ, Nodelijk G, Hagenaars TJ, Elbers ARW, de Jong MCM: Local spread of classical swine fever upon virus introduction into The Netherlands: Mapping of areas at high risk. *BMC Veterinary Research* 2008, 4:9

19. Pfeiffer DU: Geographical information science and spatial analysis in animal health.In *GIS and spatial analysis in veterinary*

science. Edited by Durr P, Gatrell A. CABI publishing, Wallingford, Oxfordshire, UK; 2004:303.

20. Anon: *Somali Livestock Statistics 1988/1989.* Ministry of Livestock, Forestry and Range - Department of Planning and Statistics, Mogadishu, Somalia;
21. Tempia S: The dynamic of Rinderpest in nomadic pastoral systems: the Somali surveillance example. *PhD thesis*. Colorado State University. Fort Collins-Colorado;
22. Anderson J, McKey JA, Butcher RN: The use of monoclonal antibodies in competitive ELISA for the detection of antibodies to rinderpest and peste des petits ruminants.In *The Sero-Monitoring of Rinderpest Through Africa - Phase I. Proceedings of the Final Research Coordination Meeting of IAEA Rinderpest Control Projects*. International Atomic Energy Agency, Vienna; 1991.
23. Africa Data Sampler: *A Geo-Referenced Database for All African Countries*. World Resources Institute in Collaboration with World Conservation Monitoring Centre and Padco, Inc. CD-ROM; 2000.
24. UNDOS: *Somalia Topomaps*. United Nations Development Office for Somalia (UNDOS), Nairobi, CD-ROM; 2003.
25. White GC, Garrott RA: *Analysis of wildlife radiotracking data*. Academic Press, New York. New York, USA; 1990.
26. Carrat F, Valleron AJ: Epidemiologic mapping using the "Kriging" method: application to an influenza-like illness epidemic in France. *American Journal of Epidemiology* 1992, 135:1293-1300.
27. Olivier MA, Webster R: Kriging: a method of interpolation for geographical information systems. *International Journal of Geographical Information Systems* 1990, 4:313-332.
28. Stein ML: *Interpolation of Spatial Data - Some Theory for Kriging*. Springer-Verlag, Inc., New York; 1999.
29. Webster R, Olivier MA, Muir KR, Mann JR: Kriging the local risk of a rare diseases from a register of diagnosis. *Geographical Analysis* 1994, 26:168-185.
30. Lessard P, L'Eplattenier R, Norval RAI, Kundert K, Dolan TT, Croze H: Geographical information systems for studying the epidemiology of cattle disease caused by Theileria parva. *The Veterinary Record* 1990, 126:255-262.

31. Cressie NAC: *Statistics for spatial data*. John Wiley & Sons, New York, USA; 1993.

32. Terra Nuova: Improvement and Diversification of Somali Livestock Trade and Marketing. Fourth Progress Report. In *August 2006 to January 2007*. Terra Nuova, Nairobi, Kenya; 2007.

33. Terra Nuova: PanAfrican Control for the Epizootics - Somali Component. Rinderpest Cross-Sectional Sero-Survey in Central and Southern Somalia-Technical Report. *Terra Nuova, Nairobi* 2003.

34. Hardin J, Hilbe J: *Generalized Linear Models and Extensions*. Stata Press, Texas. USA; 2001.

35. Zenilman JM, Ellish N, Fresia A, Glass G: The geography of sexual partnerships in Baltimore: Applications of core theory dynamics using a geographic information system. *Sex Transm Dis* 1999, 26:75-81.

36. Leenders R Th. AJ: Modeling social influence through network autocorrelation: constructing the weight matrix. *Social Networks* 2002, 24:21-47.

37. Anselin L: Specification tests on the structure of interaction in spatial econometric models. *Papers of the Regional Science Association* 1984, 54:165-182.

38. Terra Nuova: *Follow-up investigation of the rinderpest situation in central and southern Somalia*. Somali Animal Health Services Project - Technical Report, Terra Nuova, Nairobi; 2005.

39. Terra Nuova: *Participatory disease search and purposive sero-surveillance for rinderpest in central and southern Somalia*. Somali Animal Health Services Project - Technical Report, Terra Nuova, Nairobi; 2006.

40. Terra Nuova: *Rinderpest cross-sectional sero-survey in the Somali Eco-System: Somalia component*. Somali Animal Health Services Project - Technical Report, Terra Nuova, Nairobi; 2006.

41. African Union-Interafrican Bureau for Animal Resources (AU-IBAR): *Rinderpest situation in the Somali Eco-System*. AU-IBAR, Nairobi; 2006.

Chapter 9

Socio-Economic Impact of Rift Valley Fever to Pastoralists and Agro Pastoralists in Arusha, Manyara and Morogoro Regions in Tanzania

Augustino A Chengula[1], Robinson H Mdegela[2], and Christopher J Kasanga[1]

[1]Department of Veterinary Microbiology and Parasitology, Faculty of Veterinary Medicine, Sokoine University of Agriculture, Morogoro, Tanzania

[2]Department of Veterinary Medicine and Public Health, Faculty of Veterinary Medicine, Sokoine University of Agriculture, Morogoro, Tanzania

ABSTRACT

Rift Valley fever (RVF) is a viral notifiable zoonotic disease primarily of domestic ruminants that causes significant socio-economic impacts. Using the 2006–07 outbreak cases, this study aimed to establish the socio-economic impact of RVF and assessing knowledge, attitude and practice of livestock keepers towards controlling RVF in selected areas of Tanzania. Data were collected in Arusha, Manyara and Morogoro regions using questionnaires, focus group discussions and in-depth interviews with key informants. Results indicate that there was little knowledge on disease (all clinical signs scored <50%) and the difference between the three regions was statistically significant (P=0.00459). Socio-economic impacts of RVF shown by this study included; animal and human deaths, disruption of livestock market chains, inability of pastoralists to achieve their daily demands, inability to obtain protein leading to malnutrition and monetary loss at individual and national level during control of the disease. These findings have demonstrated low knowledge of the community on RVF, thus, more education and engagement is needed in order to develop more effective and efficient control strategies.

BACKGROUND

Rift Valley fever (RVF) is an acute vector-borne viral zoonotic disease affecting domestic animals and humans (Davies and Martin 2006). The disease is caused by the Rift Valley fever virus (RVFV), a member of the genus Phlebovirus of the family Bunyaviridae (Elliott 1997; Elliott 1990). The transmission of RVFV in domestic animals is either through bites from different species of infected mosquitoes, mainly the *Aedes* and *Culex* genera or by direct contact with infected animal tissues, bodily fluids and fomites, particularly if associated with abortions (Davies and Martin 2006; Soti et al. 2013). Transmission of the virus to humans is thought to occur by arthropod vectors, aerosols of blood or amniotic fluid, or other direct contact with infected animals (Woods et al. 2002). The relative importance of each mode of transmission varies according to the stage of the epizootic: in the first stage, the bites of infected mosquitoes are the predominant mode of transmission whereas direct contact of animals with infected tissues (foetal or otherwise) may become predominant during the amplification stage of the epizootic (Pepin et al. 2010). In East Africa species which have been tested positive for RVFV using RT-PCR are *Aedes mcintoshi/circumluteolus, Aedes ochraceus, Aedes vexans, Aedes pembaensis, Aedes Pembaensis, Culex poicilipes, Culex bitaeniorhynchus; Culex quinquefasciatus, Culex univittatus, Cx. univittatus, Cx. Bitaeniorhynchus, Anopheles squamosus, Mansonia uniformis;* and *Mansonia africana* (Logan et al. 1991; Sang et al. 2010). Mosquito species identified to transmit RVFV in other parts of Africa include *Aedes juppi, Ae. caballus,* and *Ae. Linneatopennis* in South Africa (Métras et al. 2013),*Culex pipiens, Aedes vexans, Ae. Ochraceus* and *Ae. Dalzieli* in West Africa (Fontenille et al. 1998; Zeller et al. 1997). Even though the distribution of these vectors differ from one part of Africa to the other, they all use the same type of breeding sites and also feed on domestic ruminants.

The Rift Valley fever virus is thought to be maintained in nature at least in part by trans-ovarial transmission in flood water by Aedes mosquitoes during excess rainfall leading to floods referred to as '*dambos*' (Dighe et al. 2010; Jost et al. 2010; LaBeaud et al. 2007). In turn, it results into an abundance of vector mosquito species (Breiman et al. 2008). Elfadil et al. (2006) showed a positive association between RVF outbreaks and a dense mosquito population, high rainfall and the presence of lakes and/or ponds. Between epidemic waves, RVF virus circulates at very low incidence without noticeable clinical manifestation, neither in human nor in animals (FAO EMPRES WATCH 2007). Rift Valley fever epidemics have been observed at irregular intervals of about 5–20 years (FAO EMPRES WATCH 2007; Ibrahim et al. 2008). Early entomological field investigations of the virus or increased activity of virus in the vector population is one of the key element in controlling RVF (Hall et al. 2012). In East Africa, RVF outbreaks are known to be closely associated with heavy rainfall events (Soti et al. 2012). Therefore, the prediction of RVF occurrence should be accompanied by satellite measurements of global and regional elevated sea surface temperatures, elevated rainfall, and satellite derived-normalized difference vegetation index data (Anyamba et al. 2010). Also the assumed importance of temporary ponds and rainfall temporal distribution especially during inter-epidemic periods needs to be investigated for effective control strategies of the vectors. Currently the inter-epidemic infection of RVFV in domestic animals is increasingly being reported in different parts of Africa which in most cases passes undetected (Heinrich et al.2012; Sumaye et al. 2013).

The movement of domestic animals on the other hand has been reported to facilitate the transmission of RVFV from one place to the other during the epidemics and inter-epidemics. The appearance of RVF outside the African continent (Saud Arabia and Yemen in 2000) is said to be due to animal trade movements (Balkhy and Memish 2003; Ibrahim et al. 2008; Jansen van Vuren and Paweska 2009). Therefore, the movements of animals during epidemics should be restricted to prevent the spread of RVF to uninfected areas.

RVF causes storm abortions in pregnant animals and a high mortality approaching 100% in young animals (FAO 2000; Ikegami and Makino 2009). Sheep are more susceptible with more effect than in other ruminants (Elfadil et al. 2006). In humans, RVF causes a severe influenza-like illness characterized by fever (37.8–40°C), headache, muscular pain, vomiting and extreme weight loss (FAO 2000; Mohamed et al. 2010) with mortality rate less than 2% (LaBeaud et al. 2008). The effects of infections on human health are usually greatest on herdsmen and farm workers who live in close proximity to their animals, veterinarians, abattoir workers and butchers as an occupational hazard by direct handling of infected animals and their products (Isaäcson 2001).

In Tanzania the 2006–07 RVF outbreak was reported to the Arusha Veterinary Investigation Centre (VIC) on 21st January 2007 by the District Veterinary Officer (DVO) in Ngorongoro District who observed an abnormal disease in the district with massive abortions and deaths in animals suspecting to be RVF. Copies were sent to the Director of Veterinary Services (DVS) in Dar es Salaam, Regional administrative secretary (Arusha) and to the District Council Executive Director (Loliondo). This official report was followed by the local investigations done by the DVO. Reported cases from the livestock keepers in the district were after observing cases of abortions that started in December 2006 during rainy season. After epidemiological and clinical investigations by the veterinary district office, areas which had massive abortions and deaths in animals included; Pinyinyi, Monic, Engaresero, Matale A and B, and Malambo in Ngorongoro district. The first three villages lie along the floor of the Rift Valley along shores of Lake Natron (594–637 m above sea level) while Malambo and Matale A and B villages are on the escarpment of the Rift Valley. All the affected villages had heavy rainfall that started in December 2006. Engaresero village was also the first area to report RVF in 1998 outbreak. A team of experts from the Veterinary Investigation Centre (Arusha) were sent in the suspected areas in the district to carry out investigations and to collect specimens from suspected clinical cases of RVF. Specimens were dispatched to Onderstepoort Veterinary Institute, South Africa and at Tanzania Veterinary Laboratory Agency (Tanzania) where both laboratories confirmed RVF based on samples submitted. Apart from Arusha, there were other areas in the country that at the same time were reporting unusual abortion cases in sheep and goats. These areas included Manyara, Kilimanjaro, Tanga, Dodoma, Iringa and Morogoro regions reporting cases at different time intervals. The first two human RVF suspected cases were admitted on 28th January 2007 at Mount Meru hospital being from Terrat (Simanjiro district) and Makuyuni (Monduli district) in Manyara region. Sadly both of them died on 31st January 2007. Samples from these two patients were carefully collected and sent for detailed diagnosis to the Centres for Disease Control and Prevention (CDC) laboratory in Nairobi, Kenya and both were confirmed to be positive for RVF. Rift Valley fever was officially declared to the community in the country and OIE on February 7 and 12, 2007 respectively. In Tanzania, by the end of the outbreak in July 2007 it affected 10 of 21 regions of the country and 25 of 126 districts (Ibrahim et al. 2008; Swai and Schoonman 2009). There were 144 deaths of people out of 511 suspected cases (28.1% case fatality rate), whereby 186 (36.4%) were confirmed through laboratory tests and 124 (24%) classified as probable cases (Mohamed et al. 2010).

RVF remains to be a threat to livestock keepers and nations where the disease is occurring due to its major economic implications through the costs of the measures taken at individual, collective and international levels in order to prevent or control infection and disease outbreaks Otte (2004). However, there are few studies that have examined the socio-economic effects of the past outbreaks of RVFV, which reflects a lack of research focus on the broader social effects of the disease (Dar and McIntyre 2013). The socio-economic impacts, caused by morbidity and mortality of livestock and disruption of livelihoods, markets, and the meat industry that resulted into a ban of livestock slaughter and export of animals and animal products in Tanzania were not studied thoroughly during the 2006–07 outbreaks. Thus, the main aim of this study was to establish the socio-economic impact of RVF and assess knowledge, attitudes and practices to RVF control practices in selected areas of Tanzania using the 2006–07 outbreaks as a case study. Since natural outbreaks of RVF disease are sporadic, explosive with a very small window to allow effective planning and proper management of the disease during the outbreaks, the information obtained in this study will help the government to design preparedness programmes for effective control strategies for RVF disease. This in turn will impact positively on the livelihoods of livestock keepers who either depend on sales of live animals in the pastoral areas or those who keep dairy cattle and lose milk revenue whenever there is an outbreak of RVF.

RESULTS

Socio-Economic Activities and Benefits

In this study, 15 households reported to be purely pastoralists and 59 to be agro-pastoralists and their main sources of income being livestock keeping 73 (98.6%), agriculture 58 (78.4%), business 18 (24.3%) and employment 26 (35.1%). The categories of livestock kept by majority of households in the area are cattle, goats, sheep and chickens and those kept by minority are donkeys, pigs, dogs and cats (Table 1). Pastoralists were found to keep cattle, goats, sheep and donkeys, while animals kept by agro-pastoralists in additional to those kept by pastoralists included chickens, pigs, dogs and cats. In this study 67.6% of the respondents reported to have inherited animals from their livestock keeping families.

Table 1: The total number of different animal categories and the average number kept per household in the study households

Animal category	Total number of animals	Average number kept per household	
		Pastoralist	Agro-pastoralist
Cattle	6 234	64	20
Goats	4967	52	15
Sheep	3997	43	11

Donkeys	31	0.8	0.04
Chickens	225	0	9
Dogs	18	0	0.72
Cats	8	0	0.32
Pigs	186	0	5

Chengula *et al.*

Chengula *et al. SpringerPlus* 2013 2:549 doi:10.1186/2193-1801-2-549

Local breeds (Table 2) were kept by the majority livestock household keepers. Cattle were the domestic animals that made by far the greatest contribution to livestock-based livelihoods in the study area. In the case of agriculture, crops that were cultivated included maize, beans, banana, potatoes, rice, finger-millet, sorghum, green gram, sunflower, pigeon peas, cow peas, chick peas, cassava, onions, and vegetables. Among the mentioned sources of income, livestock keeping gave them more income 53 (71.6%) followed by agriculture 12 (16.2%), while 9 (12.2%) thought that both livestock keeping and agriculture had equal contribution to income generated.

Table 2: Type of animals kept in the study area (N=74)

Animal category	Animals kept (%)	Animals kept by majority (%)
cattle	94.6	93.2
goats	90.5	93.2
sheep	78.4	78.4
chickens	37.8	25.7
donkeys	41.9	38.5
dogs	27.0	6.80
cats	16.2	2.70
pigs	5.40	1.40

Chengula *et al.*

Chengula *et al. SpringerPlus* 2013 2:549 doi:10.1186/2193-1801-2-549

The minimum, average and maximum expenditure per month of livestock households in the study area were found to be 25 000, 120 000 and 3 000 000 Tanzanian shillings (TZS) respectively at the rate of

US$ 1 to 1500 TZS. The highest expenditure was observed in Morogoro (from a pastoralist) and the lowest being in Manyara region from an agro-pastoralist (Figure 1).

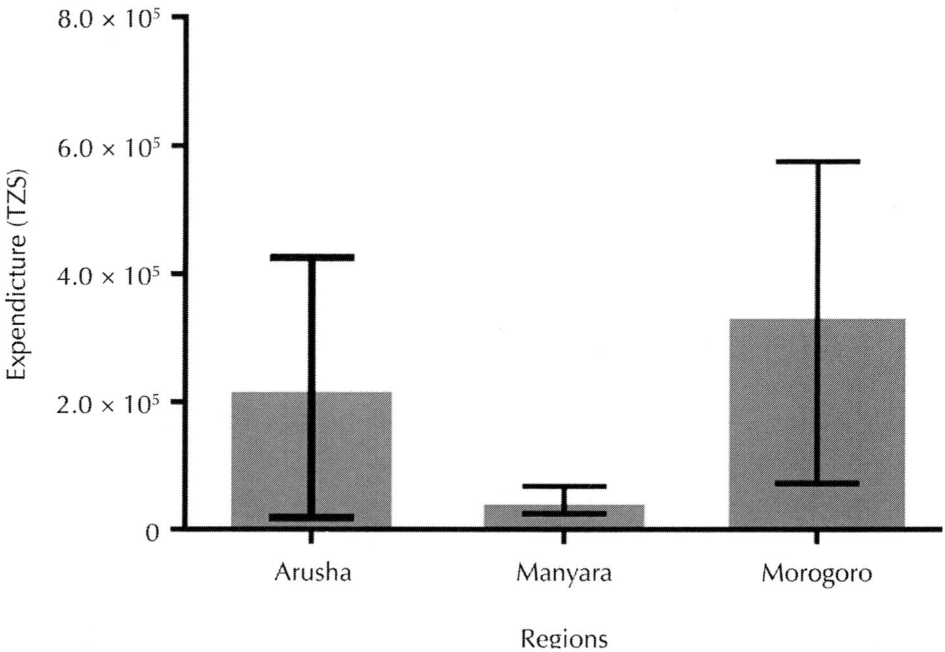

Figure 1: Representation of an average monthly expenditure of livestock households in the study area (US $1 to 1500 TZS). Expenditure levels were not significantly different between the regions (P=0.414) and within the regions (Arusha P=0.0564, Manyara P=0.0668 and Morogoro P=0.3522).

The main benefits derived from livestock keeping were reported to be food (meat, milk, ghee, and fat), socio-cultural roles such as paying dowry, school fees and buying school needs, draft power, buying household requirements and health (Table 3). Other benefits included transport for donkeys, skins, manure for crop production and building houses. Thirty (40.5%) livestock keepers used manure for crop production and the majority left it in the yard (47, 63.5%); few disposed off (11, 14.9%), sold to others (5, 6.8%) or use for decorating their houses (10, 13.5%). The amount of manure used for crop production ranged from 100 kg to 20 tonnes annually. Draught cattle were used for cultivation and or tracking luggage for an average of 3 to 5 hours per day. The average amount of milk obtained per household per day was 19.4 litres; the amount differed from one household to another depending on the number of animals kept. Only 36 (48.6%) sold their milk for a price ranging from 300 to 2000 TZS (US$ 1 to 1500 TZS). Livestock keepers earned most of their income from selling animals. The price before, during and after RVF outbreak of 2006–07 varied significantly depending on the animal species (Table 4).

Table 3: The purpose of keeping livestock as reported by livestock keepers in Arusha (n=36), Manyara (n=16) and Morogoro (n=22)

Advantage	Arusha (%)	Manyara (%)	Morogoro (%)
Paying dowry	81	44	64
School needs	97	94	95
Food	100	94	100
Agriculture	67	56	5
HHR*	100	88	100
Health care	97	81	100
Transport	25	13	5
Get manure	8	25	49

*HHR=Household requirements.

Chengula *et al.*

Chengula *et al.* *SpringerPlus* 2013 2:549 doi:10.1186/2193-1801-2-549

Table 4: Average price of selling animals before, during and after RVF outbreak of 2006-07

Animal category	Before RVF	During RVF	After RVF	P-Value	Comment
Bulls and Oxen	507 373	398 571	611 864	1.28×10-5	Significant***
Cows	328 276	267 059	40 4068	6.77×10-4	Significant**
Heifers	196 316	156 061	25 1754	1.44×10-6	Significant****
Calves	125 714	136 935	18 6786	0.0337	Significant*

Goats and sheep	40 918	36 135	61 475	1.86×10-9	Significant*****

*Indicates increasing strength of significant different in price of selling animals as the number of star increases where P>0.05 considered significant.

Chengula *et al.*

Chengula *et al. SpringerPlus* 2013 2:549 doi:10.1186/2193-1801-2-549

Livelihood Constraints

The main constraints in the area were animal diseases (Table 5), drought, inadequate pasture, water availability and lack of dipping tanks. Two (22.2%) villages during focus group discussions reported to use dipping tanks and six (66.7%) to use spray pumps to control vector borne diseases. As reported by the FGD, inadequate water and pasture in 2009 caused high mortalities in animals. Consequently, pastoralists were forced to become agro-pastoralists in northern part of Tanzania in order to cope with the losses.

Table 5: Proportion (%) of common and outbreak diseases reported in the study area by individual household (N=74)

Disease	Diseases encountered	Diseases with great loss	Diseases in outbreak form
East Coast fever	79.7	47.3	12.2
Malignant catarrhal fever	12.2	4.1	1.4
Trypanosomosis	50.0	6.8	1.4
Contagious Bovine Pleuropneumonia	45.9	24.3	13.5
Contagious Caprine Pleuropneumonia	60.8	40.5	9.5
Peste des Petits Ruminants	13.5	12.2	0.0
Rift Valley fever	2.7	0.0	36.5
Fasciolosis	10.8	4.3	0.0
Helminthosis	21.6	4.3	0.0

Anaplasmosis	17.6	6.8	1.4
Babesiosis	9.5	2.7	0.0
Anthrax	23.0	5.4	24.3
Myiasis	40.5	21.6	2.7
Foot and Mouth disease	32.4	2.7	6.8
Lumpy Skin disease	20.3	1.4	0.0
Heartwater	2.7	0.0	1.4
Black quarter	5.4	1.4	6.8
Brucellosis	0.0	0.0	1.4
Swine flue	0.0	0.0	1.4

Chengula *et al.*
Chengula *et al. SpringerPlus* 2013 2:549 doi:10.1186/2193-1801-2-549

Community Based Knowledge on Handling and Control Practices of RVF

The government used the community meetings to educate people on the presence of RVF disease in the country, how people get the disease and preventing them from eating uninspected meat. All people involved in slaughtering animals or handling slaughtered meat and livestock products were told to take all the necessary precautions. Great emphasis was given to livestock keepers to send their animals for vaccination. The community in the study area in addition received information on managing common and new diseases in the area from radio, few from LFOs and local government authorities. During the study, 69 (93.2%) reported to have heard about RVF in their life time and only 27 (36.5%) knew that it was an outbreak disease. Also 26 (35.1%) of the respondents reported that RVF disease outbreak happened in the study area and only 22 (29.7%) indicating the exact year of the last outbreak of 2006–07 with few (3, 4.1%) reporting the 1997–98 and majority failed to remember the year of the last outbreak. When asked on how RVF manifest in animals, some were able to mention the following signs; storm abortions, high fever, high mortality in lambs and kids, ocular and nasal discharge, haemorrhagic diarrhoea, vomiting, abdominal pain, jaundice and body swelling (Table 6).

Table 6: The knowledge of livestock keepers on clinical signs of RVF in livestocks in Arusha (n=36), Manyara (n=16) and Morogoro (n=22)

Clinical sign	Arusha (%)	Manyara (%)	Morogoro (%)
Storm abortions	44	19	27
High fever	28	6	0
High mortality	36	6	14
Ocular and nasal discharges	39	13	23
Haemorrhagic diarrhoea	19	0	18
Vomiting	3	0	0
Abdominal pain	6	0	0
Jaundice	25	13	14

Chengula *et al.*

Chengula *et al. SpringerPlus* 2013 2:549 doi:10.1186/2193-1801-2-549

Respondents who reported to have the disease in their household were the one who could remember significantly the clinical signs of the disease (P=0.002) and especially storm abortions, high fever, high mortality in young animals, and oculonasal discharges. On the side of the animals affected by RVF that were significantly identified in the household were goats (P=0.001) and sheep (P=0.002) probably because are the ones that were severely affected. Those who heard the disease from either neighbours, mass media, local government authority or livestock experts, most of them did not remember the clinical signs of the disease. This study has indicated that there was little knowledge on clinical signs of RVF and the difference in the three regions was statistically significant (P=0.00459).

The presence of mosquitoes in villages lying on the shores of Rift Valley especially in the evening together with floods was associated with the outbreak of the disease. Cattle, sheep, goats and human being were reported to be affected by RVF and man could get the disease from eating meat and drinking milk of RVF sick animal. Many respondents could not remember the exact year of the 2007 RVF outbreak. Livestock keepers who experienced the disease treated animals themselves using oxytetracycline, but there was no response. Respondents reported that animals were not vaccinated against RVF before the outbreak of 2006–07 as the government did not have such a control programme in their area. Livestock keepers understood that vaccination was important for controlling livestock diseases and most of them were ready to vaccinate and fully participate in the programme. During the outbreak, vaccinations were done in areas where there was no disease and targeted goats and sheep which were severely affected.

Socio-Economic Impact of RVF

The disease posed a great threat not only to the livestock keepers but also to the Government due to its social and economic implications. There were costs incurred due to measures taken at different levels in order to prevent or control infection and disease outbreaks. Rift Valley fever affected people in the study area two-fold; directly and indirectly. Directly, livestock keepers lost their animals through deaths (Tables 7 and 8) and massive abortions (Table 8), and lost all the benefits mentioned previously (Table 3).

Table 7: Status of livestock in the study households during RVF disease outbreak in the three regions

Animal category	Total No	Diseased animals	Treated animals	Animals died	Vaccinated animals
Bulls	594	37	21	21	302
Oxen	145	0	0	0	85
Cows	2398	38	38	20	1383
Heifers	403	21	21	13	248
Calves	1127	249	236	121	9
Goats	2721	128	108	50	1759
Kids	1276	205	199	164	0
Sheep	2516	49	49	35	0
Lambs	1191	133	123	119	0

Chengula *et al.*

Chengula *et al. SpringerPlus* 2013 2:549 doi:10.1186/2193-1801-2-549

Table 8: Overall deaths and abortions in domestic ruminants during the 2006/07 RVF outbreak in the study districts

		Deaths N (%)			Abortions (Total)		
Region	District	Cattle	Goat	Sheep	Cattle	Goat	Sheep
Arusha	Ngorongoro	424780 (0.29)	437103 (0.34)	327424 (0.39)	1439	1757	1314
	Longido	302272 (0.27)	391953 (0.26)	305797 (0.32)	1027	1254	1024
	Monduli	283428 (0.21)	368223 (0.20)	294395 (0.28)	776	948	847
	Arumeru	128355 (0.11)	318095 (0.05)	240915 (0.04)	143	175	101
Manyara	Simanjiro	482810 (0.10)	295883 (0.20)	148064 (0.23)	786	960	554
Morogoro	Mvomero	132560 (1.10)	98245 (1.83)	19797 (3.23)	1219	1488	559
	Kilosa	156246 (1.48)	122609 (2.33)	38542 (3.25)	1166	1423	522

Source: District veterinary offices and Veterinary Investigation Centre (Arusha). N = Total number of animals in a district, the numbers in brackets were the percent of deaths.

Chengula *et al.*

Chengula *et al. SpringerPlus* 2013 2:549 doi:10.1186/2193-1801-2-549

Non-livestock keepers were affected directly from lack of red meat as most of the markets were closed (45, 60.8%) in many areas of the country and also they were also affected by fear stress as the disease was politically exaggerated. Also indirectly non-livestock keepers were affected by competing in other sources of food which replaced the red meat such as chicken, sardines, pork, vegetables, fish and beans. The price for these replacements became high making low income people failing to buy them creating another big problem of malnutrition due to lack of protein-rich food. However, none of the respondents reported a household which stopped keeping animals because of the impact caused by RVF in the study area. Turning to agro-pastoralist was their copying strategy after the outbreak.

Reports from Tanzania Veterinary Laboratory Agency (TVLA) indicated that there were deaths of 16 973(0.10%) cattle, 20 913(0.18%) goats and 12 124(0.31%) sheep and 15 726(0.09%) abortions in cattle, 19 199(0.16%) in goats and 11 085(0.28%) in sheep. Both reports from District veterinary offices and Arusha VIC and TVLA show that sheep were highly affected followed by goats then cattle. Livestock keepers highly depends on their animals for their daily needs (Table 3), they sell their animals so that they can sustain their needs. The changes that took place during the disease in terms of price for selling animals greatly affected livestock keepers. During the RVF outbreak the average price for the different category of animals went down and became higher after the outbreak except in calves where the price increased progressively (Table 4).

Psychological Distress of Diseased Families

The livestock household that were affected by RVF in 2006–07 faced psychological distress associated with the disease. The psychological distress included loss of living confidence (fear of death), possibility of contracting the disease, possibility of losing animals as they depended on them, fear of eating meat and loss of livestock market due to legal restriction of livestock markets in and outside the country. During focus group discussion, it was reported that, not only the diseased families who appeared to experience psychological problems, but many individuals which included livestock and non-livestock keepers. Psychological distress was reported during questionnaire survey to be more severe in families that had RVF in their households. In this study, the households whose livestock had RVF were 18 (50%), 6 (38%) and 10 (45%) in Arusha, Manyara and Morogoro respectively.

Challenges for Controlling RVF Outbreaks

This study has revealed some challenges for managing animal and human disease disasters in the country. These challenges need to be addressed for effective future control RVF outbreaks. The main challenges that have been observed in this study are as follows:

Housing

Most human and animal housing in the pastoral and agro-pastoral systems in Tanzania are not reliable and more so for animals. As it was observed during the study (Figure 2), some communities had their houses at the centre of the animal's house while others were just close to the human houses and open. This was reported during in-depth interview with the key informants as one of the factors that contributed to the occurrence of the first RVF human cases in the pastoral settings as in the intensive farming systems animal houses were in good condition and well closed.

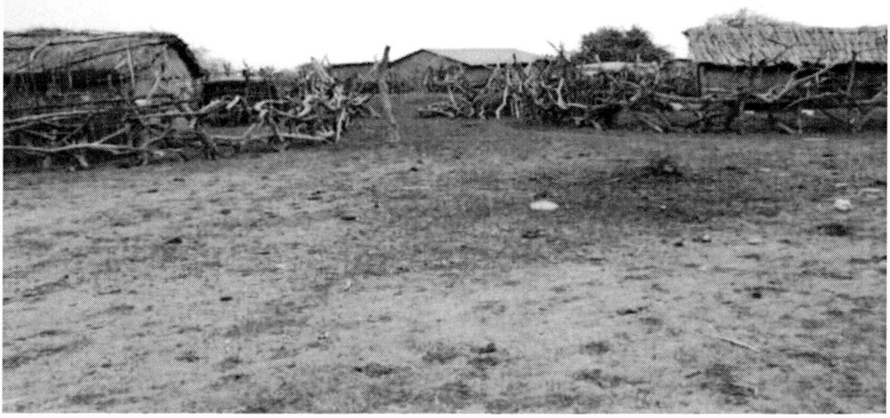

Figure 2: Representation of Maasai community village (Monic village, Ngorongoro district in Tanzania) on the Eastern arm of Rift Valley shared houses with domestic animals during the outbreak.

Inadequate Knowledge on Control Methods for RVF

This study has indicated that only 2.7% (2) of the respondents got knowledge about RVF and that 10 (13.5%) knew that there was a control measure currently in place that involved vaccination. The level of literacy in the study community was low due to nomadic lifestyle with 37.8% (28) being illiterate, 39.2% (29) standard seven, 5.4% (4) form four, and 1.4% (1) of the respondents being college graduates. This has an impact not only in the transmission and implementation of control strategies for RVF but also in the control of other livestock diseases.

Control of Animal Movements

Animal movements contribute very much on the spread of RVF from one village to another. During the 2006–07 outbreaks in Tanzania, animal movements were restricted and local government authorities reinforced regulation about animal movements. However, there were some people who moved animals from one village to another in search for pastures and water with few for search of livestock markets in near village, district, region or country (Kenya). Only five (6.8%) respondents reported to control animal movement in their households during the outbreak and they were agro-pastoralists.

Treatment of Animals by Livestock Keepers

Veterinary services in agro-pastoral and pastoral communities in Tanzania are mainly provided by LFOs who are found at least in each ward. However, provision of service to animals has been very minimal due to uncontrolled animal movements and treatment by farmers. During the outbreak of RVF in 2006–07, 17 (23%) of the households treated their animals either themselves (14, 18.9%) or LFOs (2, 2.7%). During focus group discussions, farmers said that they treated animals because it was expensive to call LFOs who demanded payments for fuel and drugs. The knowledge for treating animals by themselves was acquired from the family members and other livestock keepers. Free market economy for veterinary drugs led to easy access. Some veterinary drugs are sold in open markets (*'minada'*) sometimes in direct sun rays. These drugs came from local veterinary shops available in Tanzania and some from Kenya (farmers from the northern part). This has great impact in the control of diseases especially outbreaks as they will report after so many trials while the disease is spreading to other animals and households or villages. The main drug for treatment for many diseases in the households was Oxytetracycline (OTC). This drug was used to treat RVF cases but there was no response at all.

Consumption Habits of Meat and Milk

In pastoral and agro-pastoral communities meat inspection is not commonly practiced hence respondents reported consumption of meat without inspection as a normal practice. Both confirmed human cases in Arusha and Manyara as reported by key informants and focus groups was due to consumption of meat from dead sheep. Despite the local government authorities prohibiting people from eating meat without inspection and drinking unpasteurized milk during the outbreak, some people continued to eat meat and drink raw milk.

Insufficiency of Dipping Tanks

The use of acaricides to control ticks and other ectoparasites in the pastoral and agro-pastoral farming systems is not effective due to their nomadic life styles. Focus groups indicated that only two villages (N = 9) had dipping tanks and the remaining villages controlled ticks by spraying animals. The method of controlling ticks by spraying animals is tiresome especially for a large group of animals.

Delay on Emergency Plans for Controlling RVF

There was a complaint from some key informants that they were not involved during initial stages of preparations of emergency plans despite the fact that they knew the areas of outbreaks very well. As being experts in the areas, they could advise the government appropriately regarding important areas for vaccinations, because some vaccinations were done in areas where it was not necessary or of priority. There was a delayed response following communication with government officials. This was attributed to either long chain of command or slow acting of the responsible people (administrators) along the chain or not having emergency plan for RVF. Early warning message were issued by EMPRES in November 2006 predicting RVF outbreak in sub-Saharan Africa based on predictive climatic models like NDVI (Normal differential vegetation index), elevated temperatures in the Pacific and Indian oceans that indicated heavy rains, elevated humidity, and cloud cover favouring increased population of mosquitoes that support and spread RVF virus (FAO EMPRES WATCH 2006; Martin et al. 2007; Dijkman et al. 2009). This information was not acted upon on time in Tanzania. The disease outbreak started in late November 2006 while vaccinations started early march 2007. The human resource was available but the problem was a delay in accessing funds, equipment, and vaccines. During the outbreak, vaccines came very late and were insufficient to cover the number in infected areas. In some occasions vaccines came but there were no funds to allow vaccination campaigns to start.

Lack of Coordination and Inter-lectorial Collaboration

During in-depth interviews the key informants reported that the control of RVF was highly influenced by politicians. Vaccinations were carried out in areas which did not qualify based on vaccination regimes. In this case areas with infections could be vaccinated boosting up the disease. There was no clear mode of coordination between the central government (Ministry), and local governments (Districts) on inputs distributions. Some inputs were distributed directly to districts, some to veterinary investigation centres with no or little harmonization and coordination. The link between livestock sector and public health sector was inadequate especially on disease diagnosis and control.

Low Diagnostic Capacity

During the outbreak, samples from human being and animals were taken to Kenya and South Africa for confirmation. This caused a delay on official declaration on the presence of disease and containing the disease in the country leading to more socio-economic effects. By the time of last outbreak the country did not have a level three biosafety laboratory where tests for RVFV could be handled. Diagnosis of RVF in the country depended on clinical signs and ELISA tests at TVLA in Dar es Salaam.

DISCUSSION

Findings from this study have revealed that the majority of farmers think livestock keeping give more income than cropping. Farmers in the study area depend on livestock as the main source of income. However, diseases and drought pose serious threats to livestock keepers. Losses are attributable to morbidity, mortality and costs of disease treatment and control measures to meet national and international requirements. Epidemic diseases such as RVF, with few natural factors to limit their spread and experience in managing them bring great threat to livestock keepers. Tanzania has an estimated livestock population of 17 million cattle, 11 million goats, and 3.6 million sheep (Mohamed et al. 2010) most of which are located in the north and central regions of the country. These regions were severely affected by the 2006–07 RVF outbreak leading to disrupted socio-economic setting of all Tanzanians and more so livestock keepers who are completely dependent on livestock and their products.

The 2006–07 RVF outbreak in Tanzania started in the northern part with abnormal abortions and deaths in domestic animals in late December 2006 and confirmed in January 2007. In early February 2007, the Government of Tanzania held an emergency inter-ministerial meeting in Arusha after which the District Commissioners were given tasks to prepare strategies to control the disease in their districts. One of the strategies was to provide education to the community on clinical appearance of the disease, spread of disease (transmission) and the effect of disease to human and their animals. Also education was given in slaughter premises to all people who were involved in handling and slaughtering animals. Livestock keepers were emphasized to make sure they did not move animals from one village to another and that they were to participate fully in vaccination campaigns.

During this time the government was ordering Smithburn vaccines abroad and organizing funds and human resources. The first vaccine doses were received by the government in the end of February 2007, 116 600 were distributed to districts with reported cases namely Monduli, Ngorongoro, Simanjiro, Longido, Hai, Babati, Mkinga and Kilosa. Also equipments and funds to run vaccination campaigns were provided by the Government. Additional, 370 400 vaccine doses were distributed to all districts as well as in other two districts namely Iringa rural and Mvomero in which RVF cases were reported. Vaccination campaigns to animals started early on March 2007 to all ages of cattle, sheep and goats except those under six months and pregnant animals were vaccinated. Emphasis was put on sheep and goats when the amount of vaccine was not enough. Vaccinations started on the high risk areas for RVF and ended on the low risk areas based on the known history of RVF outbreaks.

This study has revealed that, during the outbreak minimal education was given to the community in the study area and more so to the pastoralists who live nomadic life. Pastoralists depended much on radios to get information about RVF as they can carry with them even to the remote grazing areas. The government used community meetings, posters, newspapers and seminars to educate communities. Since during this study, most of community members were found with low knowledge about RVF may imply that, the education provided was not effective. It has been reported by other researchers in Tanzania and elsewhere (Cripps 2000; Fyumagwa et al. 2011; Swai et al. 2010) that, it is not only livestock keepers, but also veterinary field staff and staff in health facilities, have a low awareness and poor knowledge of zoonoses. In livestock keeping community, the majority of them had not gone to school and therefore posters were not suitable for them. In this regard, providing education via their local leaders and radios could be the best option for livestock keeping community to get education easily during RVF outbreak. Vernacular languages should be used when providing education and information to the pastoralist as it has been seen that there was good proportion of people who could not understand and speak the national language (Kiswahili). This observation was also noted in Kenya (Munyua et al. 2010) as among obstacles for efficient dissemination of information and extension of knowledge to livestock keepers. With advancement of communication technology, the use of automated messages via mobile phones that would provide information on outbreak of diseases may be useful. Majority of the livestock keepers nowadays in Tanzania own and use mobile phones for their family matters and seeking market information. The application of mobile technologies by the livestock keepers and veterinary professionals to exchange information on livestock diseases will enhance disease surveillance (Karimuribo et al. 2011a).

During the 2006–07 RVF outbreaks, some farmers went on eating meat without inspection and proper cooking that led to more human cases especially in some parts of Dodoma. This was due to their socio-cultural behaviour of eating meat not inspected or from dead animals. This calls further educational intervention at community levels. The limited knowledge of pastoral communities on risk practices including eating raw meat, raw milk, touching and herding aborted animals and consuming products from animals predisposes them to zoonotic diseases (Anyangu et al. 2010). On the other hand in some communities it was observed that human and animals shared the same housing that also predisposed them to zoonotic diseases. This has also been observed and associated as one of the risk factor for transmitting zoonotic diseases (including RVF) to human (Jost et al. 2010; Swai et al. 2010). Hence more education is needed and interventions that will enable the community live in separate houses from animals.

In pastoral communities, animals that get sick are often treated by themselves due to unavailability of livestock disease professional and para-professionals that can take charge in disease diagnosis, treatment and other disease management. Other factors include high treatment cost linked to calls of veterinary doctors and buying of drugs, keeping large number of animals just for prestige, nomadic lifestyle and insufficient knowledge on best ways to control diseases. Apart from livestock experts being few, nomadic lifestyle contributes by far for the limited access to veterinary services that would provide service on time. Pastoralists have limited knowledge about dosage and routes for drug administration. Free market economy for veterinary pharmaceutical in Tanzania contributes greatly to self-treatment of animals by and mishandling of drugs. Easy access to drugs and self-treatment procedures have great impact on control of livestock diseases especially during outbreaks as pastoralists will report after so many trials, while the disease is progressing to spread. The use of trained Community Animal Health Workers (CAHWs) as an important alternative animal to animal health delivery channel in the country's marginal areas where there are few professional veterinary practitioners will help to reduce the problems (Allport et al. 2005; Swai and Masaaza 2012). In the rural settings health delivery systems are hampered by many factors including remoteness, poor infrastructure, inadequate transport, lack of qualified veterinary staffs and insufficient funds to support surveillance operations and buy reagents and drugs (Swai and Schoonman 2012). Therefore, the use of CAHWs could be a good link to the veterinary professionals and the livestock disease control units for providing information to the livestock keepers and to the veterinary experts.

During the outbreak, the quarantine was not executed properly as pastoralists could still move their animals from one village to another to search for pastures. Also farmers were still selling animals to nearby country (Kenya) via unauthorized routes. The movement of animals from Tanzania to Kenya either for search of good pasture or for sale has been reported (Diallo et al.2000) to facilitate further spread of the disease to unaffected areas during the 2006–07 RVF outbreak. It was observed that good pastures were found in the low land areas where mosquitoes were also found in large numbers and facilitated the disease transmission. However, the short difference in time of occurrence of disease in different regions of Tanzania is an indication that, those foci of outbreaks were caused by other factors other than animal movement as it was also highlighted by (FAO 2000). The results also indicated that few farmers used dipping tanks and the majority used spray pumps to control vector borne diseases. Since some of the farmers owned large number of animals, it was not possible to effectively spray all of them. According to (Peter et al. 2005) and (Davies and Martin 2006) effective use of dipping tanks also reduces the magnitude of mosquito borne diseases like RFV.

Rift Valley fever led to disruption of whole market chains system in the country similar to what it was reported in other countries that experienced the disease (Holleman 2002). The study has indicated that sheep were highly affected followed by goats then cattle as it was observed in Kenya (Jost et al. 2010) following similar outbreaks. This was contributed by lack of emergency plans that led to delayed control of RVF in the country. This was a similar observation in Kenya (FAO EMPRES WATCH 2006; Martin et al. 2007). Thus, there is a need of having organizational rearrangement so that an emergency unit is put in place that will deal with emergency diseases especially outbreaks or unknown cases that require fast action to prevent massive socio-economic loses. The normal administrative structures of national veterinary services that deals with routines animal health programmes have been reported (FAO 2000) to be ineffective for emergency cases. During the 2006–07 RVF outbreak in Tanzania, the coordination for controlling the disease was under the umbrella of the National Disaster Preparedness and Response unit within the Prime Minister's Office (Karimuribo et al. 2011b). Establishment of the unit will ensure active surveillance and monitoring is carried out routinely in the field to create baseline information on inter-epidemic virus transmission patterns, areas at risk and early warning of RVFV activity or increased mosquito populations. Also annual vaccinations in highly susceptible areas identified by experienced livestock stakeholders are done together with early distribution of enough vaccine doses, equipments and funds during outbreaks.

Control measures that were put in place by the government could not be implemented properly because time frame for the disease to spread in a wider area was very short to enable the government to provide education as fast as possible. Inadequate numbers of livestock disease experts in the livestock keeping community led to livestock keepers treat their animals. This led to delayed reporting of the disease outbreaks. Also lack of collaboration between and within the livestock sectors led to difficulties in effective implementing control measures during the outbreak. Thus, there is high chance that the disease disappeared naturally. Since RVF affects human, domestic and wild animals and transmitted by arthropods, the approach towards its control should involve a number of government Ministries. In Tanzania the Ministries includes, the Ministry of Livestock Development and Fisheries, the Ministry of Health and Social Welfare and the Ministry of Natural Resources and Tourism. During the 2006/07 RVF outbreak, the Ministries responsible for Livestock Development and worked in isolation and in ad hoc manner using Ministerial contingency plans which also have no common point of intersection (Fyumagwa et al. 2011; Mbugi et al. 2012). There is a need of creating a point of intersection in order to be able to fit in the concept of 'One Health Approach' which is thought to be a better way of combating infectious diseases. The initiatives towards the One Health infectious diseases surveillance in Tanzania has been started by introducing Masters in One Health Molecular Biology at Sokoine University of Agriculture under the Southern African Centre for Infectious Diseases Surveillance (SACIDS). The Government of Tanzania launched officially the One Health Approach in Arusha on April 16, 2013 by the Vice President of the United Republic of Tanzania.

CONCLUSIONS

Rift Valley fever is a multi-disciplinary disease which demands a one heath approach in order to control it during the outbreaks. Much is needed and can be done by education, and in particular by increasing the awareness of different health professionals, and facilitating communication and collaboration between veterinary, public health and agricultural personnel on RVF. To achieve this, there must be a point of intersection in the Ministerial policies, Acts and Contingency plans that tries to address how to deal with zoonotic diseases. There is a need of establishing active surveillance system for RVFV which will capture the increase of virus activity in the vectors together with the use of other weather monitoring station (the forecast models) like the NASA Meteorological information. Annual vaccinations of domestic animals especially in areas known to be the hotspots of RVF outbreaks should be done. These should not wait for the outbreak to occur because there is very small window to prepare before the disease spreads to a wider area leading to tremendous effects.

MATERIALS AND METHODS

Study Area

The study was carried out in Arusha and Manyara where pastoral farming is practiced and Morogoro where dairy and agro pastoral farming systems are practiced in Tanzania (Figure 3). Arusha, Manyaara and Morogoro have an altitude ranging from 482 to1368 m above sea level and are among the areas that experienced RVF outbreaks in 2006–07. These areas normally experience two rainy seasons: a short rainy season between October and December, and a long rainy season between March and May. Typically, the annual precipitation averages between 500 and 1000 mm. The vegetation consists mainly of various shrubs and acacia bushes, and livestock species kept are primarily cattle, goats and sheep.

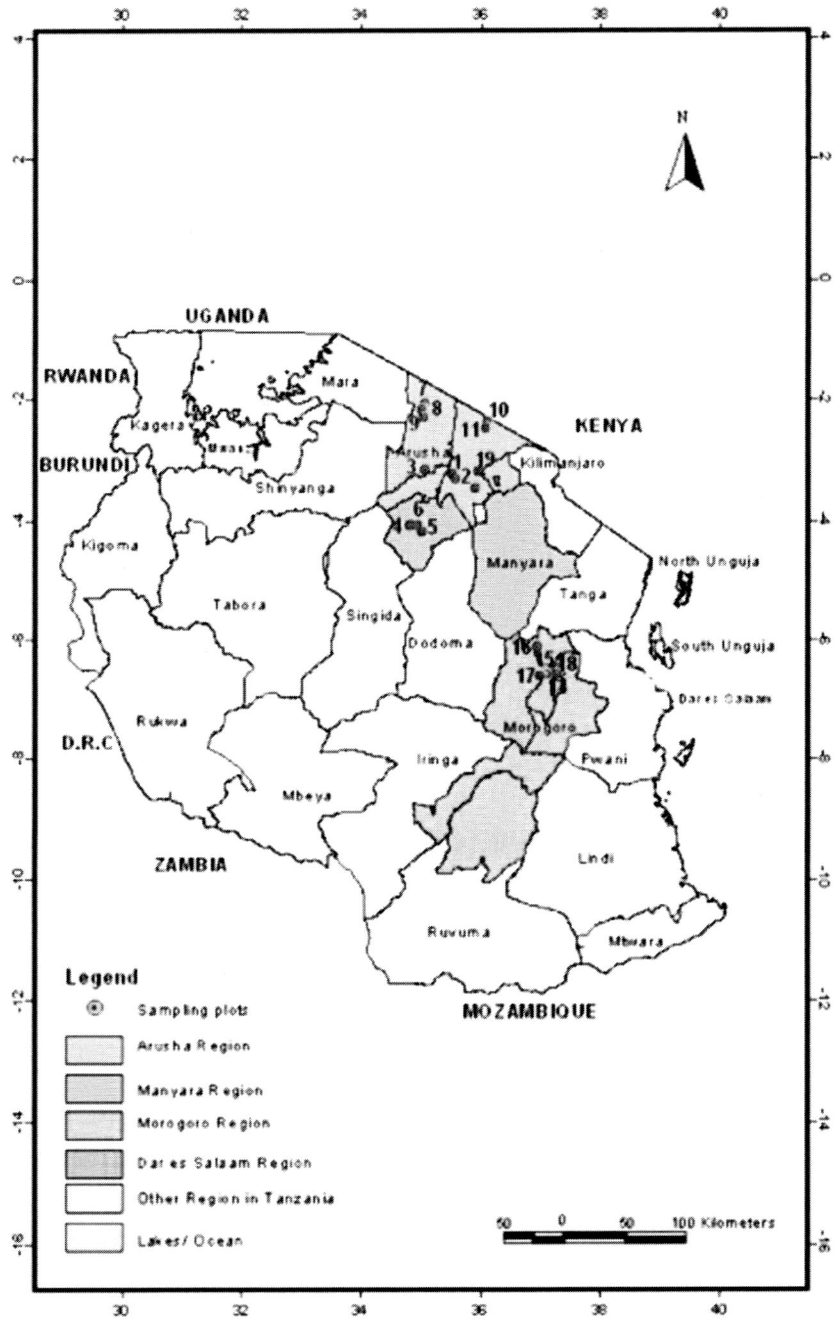

Figure 3: Representation of the map of Tanzania showing study areas: number 1 to 19 shows locations where socio-economic study was conducted in Arusha, Manyara and Morogoro regions.

Research Design

A cross-sectional study design that allows data to be collected at a single point in time was used in this study to collect data between January and April, 2012. The following formula for sample size estimation as proposed by Naing and his colleagues (2006) was used for socio-economic study;

$$n = \frac{Z^2P(1-P)}{d^2} \qquad (1)$$

Where n = estimated sample size, Z = Z statistic for 95% confidence interval (1.96), P = expected proportion of livestock household keepers with knowledge on RVF (13%) based on findings by (Labeaud et al. 2008) and d = is the margin of error set at 95% (5%). This gave a total number of 174 livestock household keepers.

Sampling Technique

In this study a multi stage sampling method was employed. A purposive sampling method was used to obtain regions based on pastoral (Arusha and Manyara regions), dairy and agro pastoral (Morogoro region) farming systems. Also these are areas which were affected by the 2006/07 RVF outbreak. The villages (19) included in this study were drawn randomly using random number generator built in Microsoft Excel 2010 from a frame of all villages in the three regions. Individual households within the villages were selected based on keeping livestock and having kept animals for more than ten years. Before commencement of the study, the questionnaires were pre tested to check the validity and how the individuals could understand and respond to questions. The questionnaires were modified on the basis of the result of the pre-test. The pre-test used a total of ten (10) livestock households in one village (Sokoine in Mvomero district) with five (5) households being pastoralists and five (5) households being agro pastoralists.

Data Collection

During the study, quantitative data were collected using questionnaire while qualitative data were collected using in-depth interviews with key informants and focus group discussions. The questionnaire was pre-tested in six farms, three for each pastoralists and agro-pastoralists.

Quantitative Data

The questionnaire survey used 74 respondents with age ranging from 21–79 years old. The participants were interviewed on socio-economic and cultural activities, type of livestock kept and livestock involvements regarding RVF disease impact on household livelihood activities. The seasonality of both human and livestock RVF issues, trade and marketing in livestock, their product and their perception on the occurrence of RVF on their livelihoods were assessed. The study determined the social organization of production; livelihood constraints; household's income sources and average monthly expenditure; number of livestock-holding households and stock of livestock in the households including data on number, species and breeds as well as the quantity of livestock products (milk, meat, manure, traction power) produced and marketed by livestock keeping households through the year. Furthermore the community based knowledge for management of RVF was established to explore on what the community know and what was implemented during the 2006–07 outbreak. The interviews also collected descriptions of the clinical presentation of RVF in people and livestock, as well as its incidence relative to other diseases.

Qualitative Data

These were general information about livestock diseases (disease outbreaks, specific view on RVF disease, control, and its significance to livestock, and government involvement to control of RVF). Also issues on livestock regulations and reasons for success and failure to implement recommended management procedures were explored during in-depth interviews. In-depth interviews were conducted with district veterinarians, veterinary investigation centre officers and LFOs who had been involved in the management of the 2006–07 outbreaks.

The study also used focus group discussions (FGD) with agro-pastoralists and pastoralists in some villages where questionnaire was administered. The focus groups involved between 5 to 12 people, most of whom were men and most were ethnically Maasai with few Mbulu, Barbaig and other tribes. Nine focus groups (three from each region) were conducted. The groups were introduced to the research topic before starting the discussion and the duration of discussion was between 30 and 60 minutes. The discussion was guided by a set of prepared questions and the permission to document and record the discussion was obtained from the participants. The focal group participants were interviewed on their economic and cultural activities, knowledge on the impact of livestock diseases and their management, responsibility for disease control, awareness on outbreak diseases especially RVF and how the community obtain general information about outbreak of diseases.

Data from Government Offices

Information on the areas affected by RVF, total number of animals died and aborted, emergency plans and the stake holders involved during the outbreak were obtained from district and regional veterinary offices, Arusha Veterinary Investigation Centre, Tanzania Veterinary Laboratory Agency and the Ministry of Livestock Development and Fisheries.

Data Analysis

In this study, Statistical Package for Social Science (SPSS) version 17.0 was used for descriptive analysis (means, frequencies) and comparing the proportions for data collected using questionnaire. Analysis of variance (ANOVA) was used to compare means between populations. The MAXQDA 10 was used for analysis of focus group discussion transcripts.

AUTHORS' CONTRIBUTIONS

AAC have made substantial contributions to acquisition of data, analysis and interpretation of results and wrote the manuscript. RHM have made a contributions to conception and design of study and proof read the manuscript. CJK have been involved in drafting the manuscript and reading it critically and gave the final approval for the version to be published. All authors read and approved the final manuscript.

ACKNOWLEDGEMENTS

The authors gratefully acknowledge the Regional Universities Forum (RUFORUM) with headquarter in Kampala, Uganda for supporting the research of this study from proposal development to completion of study. The authors also thank the District Veterinary Officers, Veterinary Investigation Centre Officers, livestock field officers and livestock keepers for their cooperation during data collection in the study area.

REFERENCES

1. Allport R, Mosha R, Bahari M, Swai E, Catley A (2005) The use of community-based animal health workers to strengthen disease surveillance systems in Tanzania. Rev Sci Tech Int Off Epizoot 24:921-932
2. Anyamba A, Linthicum KJ, Small J, Britch SC, Pak E, de La Rocque S, Formenty P, Hightower AW, Breiman RF, Chretien J-P, Tucker CJ, Schnabel D, Sang R, Haagsma K, Latham M, Lewandowski HB, Magdi SO, Mohamed MA, Nguku PM, Reynes J-M, Swanepoel R (2010) Prediction, assessment of the Rift Valley fever activity in East and Southern Africa 2006–2008 and possible vector control strategies. Am J Trop Med Hyg 83:43-51
3. Anyangu AS, Gould LH, Sharif SK, Nguku PM, Omolo JO, Mutonga D, Rao CY, Lederman ER, Schnabel D, Paweska JT, Katz M, Hightower A, Njenga MK, Feikin DR, Breiman RF (2010) Risk factors for severe Rift Valley fever infection in Kenya, 2007. Am J Trop Med Hyg 83:14-21
4. Balkhy HH, Memish ZA (2003) Rift Valley fever: an uninvited zoonosis in the Arabian peninsula. Int J Antimicrob Agents 21:153-157
5. Breiman RF, Njenga MK, Cleaveland S, Sharif S, Mbabu M, King L (2008) Lessons from the 2006–2007 Rift Valley fever outbreak

in East Africa: implications for prevention of emerging infectious diseases. Future Virol 3:411-417

6. Cripps PJ (2000) Veterinary education, zoonoses and public health: a personal perspective. Acta Trop 76:77-80
7. Dar O, McIntyre S (2013) Rift Valley fever and a new paradigm of research and development for zoonotic disease control. Infect Dis 19:189-193
8. Davies FG, Martin V (2006) Recognizing Rift Valley fever. Vet Ital 42:31-53
9. Diallo M, Lochouarn L, Ba K, Sall AA, Mondo M, Girault L, Mathiot C (2000) First isolation of the Rift Valley fever virus from Culex poicilipes (Diptera: Culicidae) in nature. Am J Trop Med Hyg 62:702-704
10. Dighe NS, Pattan SR, Bhawar SB, Gaware VM, Hole MB, Waman S, Butle SR (2010) Rift Valley fever: a review. J Chem Pharm Res 2:228-239
11. Dijkman J, Hall A, Steglich M, Sones K (2009) Innovation response capacity in relation to livestock-related emergencies in Africa (03). 1-74 Retrieved from http://www.igad-lpi.org/publication/docs/IGADLPI_WP03_10.pdf
12. Elfadil AA, Hassab-Allah KA, Dafa-Allah OM (2006) Factors associated with rift valley fever in south-west Saudi Arabia. Rev Sci Tech 25:1137-1145
13. Elliott RM (1990) Review article molecular biology of the Bunyaviridae. J Gen Virol 71:501-522
14. Elliott RM (1997) Minireview emerging viruses: the Bunyaviridae. Mol Med 3:572-577
15. FAO (2000) Emergency preparedness planning rift valley fever. Rift Val fever Man 1–10. http://www.fao.org/ag/againfo/resources/documents/AH/RVF198.htm Accessed 02 September, 2013
16. FAO EMPRES WATCH (2006) Possible RVF activity in the Horn of Africa. 1-7 http://ftp.fao.org/docrep/fao/011/aj218e/aj218e00.pdf Accessed 27 Sptember, 2013
17. FAO EMPRES WATCH (2007) Rift Valley fever could spread with movement of animals from East Africa. 1-5 http://ftp.fao.org/docrep/fao/011/aj215e/aj215e00.pdf Accessed 29 August, 2013

18. Fontenille D, Traore-Lamizana M, Diallo M, Thonnon J, Digoutte JP, Zeller HG (1998) New vectors of Rift Valley fever in West Africa. Emerg Infect Dis 4:289-293
19. Fyumagwa RD, Ezekiel MJ, Nyaki A, Mdaki ML, Katale ZB (2011) Response to Rift Valley fever in Tanzania: challenges and opportunities. Tanzan J Health Res 13:1-9
20. Hall RA, Blitvich BJ, Johansen CA, Blacksell SD (2012) Advances in arbovirus surveillance, detection and diagnosis. J Biomed Biotechnol 2012:512969 doi:10.1155/2012/512969
21. Heinrich N, Saathoff E, Weller N, Clowes P, Kroidl I, Ntinginya E, Machibya H, Maboko L, Löscher T, Dobler G, Hoelscher M (2012) High seroprevalence of Rift Valley fever and evidence for endemic circulation in Mbeya region, Tanzania, in a cross-sectional study. PLoS Negl Trop Dis 6:e1557 doi: 10.1371/journal.pntd.0001557
22. Holleman CF (2002) The socio-economic implications of the livestock Ban in Somaliland. Famine early warning system new task order2. http://pdf.usaid.gov/pdf_docs/PNADJ083.pdf Accessed on 29 September 2013
23. Ibrahim M, Aziz A, Eid-ul-adha H (2008) A post card from uk rift valley fever: the story unfolds to family in Sudan. Sudan J Public Heal 3:5-10
24. Ikegami T, Makino S (2009) Rift valley fever vaccines. Vaccine 27(Suppl 4):69-72
25. Isaäcson M (2001) Viral hemorrhagic fever hazards for travelers in Africa. Clin Infect Dis 33:1707-1712
26. Jansen van Vuren P, Paweska JT (2009) Laboratory safe detection of nucleocapsid protein of Rift Valley fever virus in human and animal specimens by a sandwich ELISA. J Virol Methods 157:15-24
27. Jost CC, Nzietchueng S, Kihu S, Bett B, Njogu G, Swai ES, Mariner JC (2010) Epidemiological assessment of the Rift Valley fever outbreak in Kenya and Tanzania in 2006 and 2007. Am J Trop Med Hyg 83:65-72
28. Karimuribo ED, Sayalel K, Beda E, Short N, Wambura P, Mboera LG, Kusiluka LJM, Rweyemamu MM (2011a) Towards One Health disease surveillance: The Southern African Centre for Infectious Disease Surveillance approach. Onderstepoort J Vet 79(2):1-7

29. Karimuribo ED, Mboera LEG, Mbugi E, Simba A, Fredrick M (2011b) Are we prepared for emerging and re-emerging diseases? Experience and lessons from epidemics that occurred in Tanzania during the last five decades. Tanzan J Health Res 13:1-14

30. LaBeaud AD, Ochiai Y, Peters CJ, Muchiri EM, King CH (2007) Spectrum of Rift Valley fever virus transmission in Kenya: insights from three distinct regions. Am J Trop Med Hyg 76:795-800

31. LaBeaud AD, Muchiri EM, Ndzovu M, Mwanje MT, Muiruri S, Peters CJ, King CH (2008) Interepidemic Rift Valley fever virus seropositivity, northeastern Kenya. Emerg Infect Dis 14:1240-1246

32. Logan TM, Linthicum KJ, Davies FG, Binepal YS, Roberts CR (1991) Isolation of Rift Valley fever virus from mosquitoes (Diptera: Culicidae) collected during an outbreak in domestic animals in Kenya. J Med Entomol 28:293-295

33. Martin V, De Simone L, Lubroth J, Ceccato P, Chevalier V (2007) Perspectives on using remotely-sensed imagery in predictive veterinary epidemiology and global early warning systems. Geospat Health 2:3-14

34. Mbugi EV, Kayunze KA, Katale BZ, Kendall S, Good L, Kibik GS, Keyyu JD, Godfrey-Faussett P, van Helden P, Matee MI (2012) "One Health" infectious diseases surveillance in Tanzania: Are we all on board the same flight? Onderstepoort J Vet 79(2):1-7

35. Métras R, Baguelin M, Edmunds WJ, Thompson PN, Kemp A, Pfeiffer DU, Collins LM, White RG (2013) Transmission potential of Rift Valley fever virus over the course of the 2010 epidemic in South Africa. Emerg Infect Dis 19:916-924

36. Mohamed M, Mosha F, Mghamba J, Zaki SR, Shieh W-J, Paweska J, Omulo S, Gikundi S, Mmbuji P, Bloland P, Zeidner N, Kalinga R, Breiman RF, Njenga MK (2010) Epidemiologic and clinical aspects of a Rift Valley fever outbreak in humans in Tanzania, 2007. Am J Trop Med Hyg 83:22-27

37. Munyua P, Murithi RM, Wainwright S, Githinji J, Hightower A, Mutonga D, Macharia J, Ithondeka PM, Musaa J, Breiman RF, Bloland P, Njenga MK (2010) Rift Valley fever outbreak in livestock in Kenya, 2006–2007. Am J Trop Med Hyg 83:58-64

38. Otte (2004) Transboundary animal diseases: assessment of socio-economic impacts and institutional responses. FAO, Livestock Policy Discussion Paper 9. http://www.fao.org/ag/againfo/resources/en/publications/sector_discuss/PP_Nr9_Final. Accessed on 29 September, 2013
39. Pepin M, Bouloy M, Bird BH, Kemp A, Paweska J (2010) Rift Valley fever virus (Bunyaviridae: Phlebovirus): an update on pathogenesis, molecular epidemiology, vectors, diagnostics and prevention. Vet Res 41:61
40. Peter RJ, Van den Bossche P, Penzhorn BL, Sharp B (2005) Tick, fly, and mosquito control lessons from the past, solutions for the future. Vet Parasitol 132:205-215
41. Sang R, Kioko E, Lutomiah J, Warigia M, Ochieng C, O'Guinn M, Lee JS, Koka H, Godsey M, Hoel D, Hanafi H, Miller B, Schnabel D, Breiman RF, Richardson J (2010) Rift Valley fever virus epidemic in Kenya, 2006/2007: the entomologic investigations. Am J Trop Med Hyg 83:28-37
42. Soti V, Tran A, Degenne P, Chevalier V, Lo Seen D, Thiongane Y, Diallo M, Guégan J-F, Fontenille D (2012) Combining hydrology and mosquito population models to identify the drivers of Rift Valley fever emergence in semi-arid regions of West Africa. PLoS Negl Trop Dis 6:e1795 doi: 10.1371/journal.pntd.0001795
43. Soti V, Chevalier V, Maura J, Bégué A, Lelong C, Lancelot R, Thiongane Y, Tran A (2013) Identifying landscape features associated with Rift Valley fever virus transmission, Ferlo region, Senegal, using very high spatial resolution satellite imagery. Int J Health Geogr 12:10 doi: 10.1186/1476-072X-12-10
44. Sumaye RD, Geubbels E, Mbeyela E, Berkvens D (2013) Inter-epidemic transmission of Rift Valley fever in livestock in the Kilombero River Valley, Tanzania: a cross-sectional survey. PLoS Negl Trop Dis 7:e2356 doi: 10.1371/journal.pntd.0002356
45. Swai E, Masaaza S (2012) Where there is no conventional veterinary health delivery services what are the capabilities of community animal health workers? Livest Res Rural Dev 24: Retrieved from http://www.lrrd.cipav.org.co/lrrd24/7/swai24114.htm
46. Swai ES, Schoonman L (2009) Prevalence of rift valley fever immunoglobulin g antibody in various occupational groups

before the 2007 outbreak in tanzania. VectorBorne Zoonotic Dis 9:579-582

47. Swai E, Schoonman L (2012) A survey of zoonotic diseases in trade cattle slaughtered at Tanga city abattoir: a cause of public health concern. Asian Pac J Trop Biomed 2:55-60
48. Swai E, Schoonman L, Daborn C (2010) Knowledge and attitude towards zoonoses among animal health workers and livestock keepers in Arusha and Tanga, Tanzania. Tanzania J Heal 12:282-288
49. Woods CW, Karpati AM, Grein T, McCarthy N, Gaturuku P, Muchiri E, Dunster L, Henderson A, Khan AS, Swanepoel R, Bonmarin I, Martin L, Mann P, Smoak BL, Ryan M, Ksiazek TG, Arthur RR, Ndikuyeze A, Agata NN, Peters CJ (2002) An outbreak of Rift Valley fever in Northeastern Kenya, 1997–98. Emerg Infect Dis 8:138-144
50. Zeller HG, Fontenille D, Traore-Lamizana M, Thiongane Y, Digoutte JP (1997) Enzootic activity of Rift Valley fever virus in Senegal. Am J Trop Med Hyg 56:265-272

Citations

CHAPTER 1

Gabriele Volpato and Patricia Howard, The material and cultural recovery of camels and camel husbandry among Sahrawi refugees of Western Sahara, doi: 10.1186/s13570-014-0007-4.

CHAPTER 2

Jimmy T. Efird, tephen W. Davies, Wesley T. O'Neal, and Ethan J. Anderson, Animal Viruses, Bacteria, and Cancer: A Brief Commentary, doi: 10.3389/fpubh.2014.00014.

CHAPTER 3

R. Chazya, J. B. Muma, K. K. Mwacalimba, E. Karimuribo, E. Mkandawire, and M. Simuunza, "A Qualitative Assessment of the Risk of Introducing Peste des Petits Ruminants into Northern Zambia from Tanzania,"Veterinary Medicine International, vol. 2014, Article ID 202618, 10 pages, 2014. doi:10.1155/2014/202618.

CHAPTER 4

Barend Mark de Clare Bronsvoort, Samuel Mwangi Thumbi, Elizabeth Jane Poole, Henry Kiara, Olga Tosas Auguet, Ian Graham Handel, Amy Jennings, Ilana Conradie, Mary Ndila Mbole-Kariuki, Philip G Toye, Olivier Hanotte, JAW Coetzer, and Mark EJ Woolhouse, Design and descriptive epidemiology of the Infectious Diseases of East African Livestock (IDEAL) project, a longitudinal calf cohort study in western Kenya, DOI: 10.1186/1746-6148-9-171.

CHAPTER 5

Katharina DC Stärk, Gertraud Regula, Jorge Hernandez, Lea Knopf, Klemens Fuchs, Roger S Morris, and Peter Davies, Concepts for Risk-Based Surveillance in the Field of Veterinary Medicine and Veterinary Public Health: Review of Current Approaches, doi:10.1186/1472-6963-6-20.

CHAPTER 6

Heiko Nathues, Johanna Meyer-Hamme, Petra Maass, Ruediger Goessl, Wibke Stansen, Rolf Steens, and Elisabeth grosse Beilage, Reliability of Operational Data from Pig Herds and Performance Ratings by Veterinarians and Pig Farmers Collected During Telephone Interviews for The Evaluation of A Pcv2 Piglet Vaccination, doi:10.1186/s12917-014-0260-1.

CHAPTER 7

Kerry A Woodbine, Graham F Medley, Stephen J Moore, Ana M Ramirez-Villaescusa, Sam Mason, and Laura E Green, A Four Year Longitudinal Sero-Epidemiological Study of Bovine Herpesvirus Type-1 (BHV-1) In Adult Cattle In 107 Unvaccinated Herds In South West England, doi:10.1186/1746-6148-5-5.

CHAPTER 8

Angel Ortiz-Pelaez, Dirk U Pfeiffer, Stefano Tempia, F Tom Otieno, Hussein H Aden, and Riccardo Costagli, "Risk mapping of Rinderpest sero-prevalence in Central and Southern Ssomalia based on spatial and network risk factors ", doi:10.1186/1746-6148-6-22.

CHAPTER 9

Augustino A Chengula, Robinson H Mdegela, and Christopher J Kasanga, Socio-Economic Impact of Rift Valley Fever to Pastoralists and Agro Pastoralists in Arusha, Manyara and Morogoro Regions in Tanzania, doi:10.1186/2193-1801-2-549.

Index